# BLOOD BROTHER

*a memoir*

Johnny's bone marrow could save my life,
but he'd vanished thirty years ago.

# SUSAN KELLER

TouchPoint Press
*Relax. Read. Repeat.*

BLOOD BROTHER: A MEMOIR
By Susan Keller
Published by TouchPoint Press
Brookland, AR 72417
www.touchpointpress.com

ISBN 13: 978-1-952816-39-0

TouchPoint Press books may be purchased in bulk or at special discounts for sales promotions, gifts, fundraising, or educational purposes. For details, contact the Sales and Distribution Staff: info@touchpointpress.com or via fax: 870-200-6702.

Editor: Jenn Haskin
Cover Design: Colibe Myles
Cover Images: Little Brother and Big Sister © Jamie Melton, used with permission; San Francisco Bay View © Susan Keller

First Edition

Printed in the United States of America.

*Dedicated to Dan, Elspeth, Johnny, Anne, and Dr. Greyz.*
*Without you, I would not be here.*

*And to all the family, friends, and healthcare professionals*
*who supported me every step of the way on my arduous patient journey,*
*my most sincere and lasting thanks.*

**The Full Scope of the Patient Journey**

*As a cancer survivor myself, I literally had goosebumps as I relived Susan's experience learning the seriousness of her diagnosis and prevailing through treatment. A beautiful story of the strength of the human spirit and fierce determination to live. I hope that others who have been faced with a cancer diagnosis will also find inspiration, healing, and closure in reading this most compelling memoir.*

*As a physician, I trust that other medical professionals who read* Blood Brother *will understand the full scope of the Patient Journey and the healthcare providers' powerful role within it. This book is insightful and illuminating. I highly recommend it to all readers.*

—Joanna Mimi Choi, M.D.

**Great writer, great book!**

*Thanks, and praise to Susan Keller for her extraordinary medical memoir,* Blood Brother. *Though facing a potentially fatal illness can be terrifying, it's also a priceless opportunity to learn, reconnect, and heal. Susan captures and shares these major life changes in a truly accessible way.*

*Because I'm an M.D., I picked up* Blood Brother *with a little trepidation regarding what it might disclose about us medical professionals. Because I'm also a patient with a chronic illness, I was wondering what I might discover that would be of use to me as well. What I found within were beautiful lessons, for doctor and patient alike.*

*The prognosis for Susan's particular cancer was dismal and her recovery arduous. But she presents the process with insight and even humor and joy. I also loved living through her family relationship discoveries. How our early experiences shape our later health is cutting-edge medicine today; and so, to read a cancer memoir that includes her discoveries about her brother and their early life is an extra plus for me.*

—Amy Ewing, M.D.

**THANK YOU! I am blown away.**

*I spent all day Saturday and most of the night reading* Blood Brother *and forced myself to stop at 3 AM (I just could not put it down!) It is truly an eye opener to see the whole illness process through Susan's memories and feelings, and to learn of her family story. My older son, who is captivated by medicine, is reading it and loving it too. This is a great book for anyone who treats patients, and for the patients and their families as well. It brings the Patient Journey into clear and dramatic focus.*

—Natalia Greyz, M.D.

**A Must Read for All Providers**

*From the first few engrossing pages, I was right there sharing Susan's extraordinary experiences with her.* Blood Brother *is a must read for oncologists and other providers who believe their only responsibility is to treat the patient's medical symptoms. It will inform and enrich the professional lives of those across the healthcare spectrum, adding depth and meaning to their days and producing better outcomes for patients.* Blood Brother *gives hope to those who've lost theirs, patients as well as practitioners. There are happy endings after all!*

—Meryl Luallin
CEO, SullivanLuallin Group
"Dedicated to a better care experience."

# Contents

# Prologue - January 2006

IN THE COOL WINTER SUN, I sit on a slab of limestone at the north shore of the San Francisco Bay, one long block from my home. I wait for the call from Dr. Greyz, my oncologist. The seaweed smells briny. The rocking movement of the green water comforts me. The crown of Mount Tamalpais is shrouded in clouds. It could rain tonight. In my pocket, I toy with a pewter coin inscribed with the words, "All Shall Be Well." In my other hand, my cell phone buzzes. It's Dr. Greyz.

"I am glad to have got you." Her quirky Ukrainian syntax is, as always, amusing, but her words are clipped. "The news, it is not the best."

I release the coin.

"I hate to say, but neither of your brothers' stem cells are a match."

I pull the knit wool cap farther down my bald head. This cannot be true. They'd volunteered and wanted to help. I'd assumed that one or both of them would be able to donate stem cells. There was a fifty-fifty chance. Tears well up in my eyes. Feeling shaky and vulnerable, I wrap my wool coat around me.

"And there is no one in the international database. I am very sorry."

"Can we look again? In the database?" I ask.

"If there is no one now, the chances of a match...." She pauses, then sighs.

Evening lights begin to illuminate the slate-blue skyline of San Francisco and the bridges that span the bay. Outgoing currents sweep flocks of tidal birds farther from shore. I stare at them until they become little more than specks in the restless water.

"What will we do?" I ask.

"I am so very sorry."

Without a bone marrow transplant, my chances are not good. I might not have a chance.

"I really thought…." I begin. Then, in my shock and disappointment at this shattering news, I blurt out, "I have a third brother."

"Another … another brother?" Dr. Greyz sounds stunned.

"I don't know where he is."

I am too ashamed to tell her that Johnny and I haven't spoken in decades.

And after all this time, I don't know how I feel about seeing him. There is guilt, discomfort at our years of estrangement, maybe even shame. And if I can find him, which is likely impossible, will he agree to be tested? Want to see me? Do I deserve his help?

"He could be anywhere, or nowhere," I say. "I haven't seen him in thirty years."

I struggle to stand. The tide pummels the riprap below my feet. After months of punishing chemo, I thought I'd come so far. Now, I'm back at the beginning.

"Find him. You must," says Dr. Greyz.

If I want to live, and I do, I will have to find Johnny. But how? I have no idea.

# Chapter 1 - September 2004

HOT WATER PELTS MY BACK on a stunning, late summer morning. I stretch my neck toward my chest and sigh in pleasure. I adore hot water. My soapy fingertips slide down my neck then stop at a bump a few inches under my left jaw. I press at it. Hard and painless. A jab of fear makes me frown. What is it?

Nothing clearly, just a swollen lymph gland that will quickly disappear.

Placing a hand over my obstinate, rounded belly, I push it in; it pops right out. Despite sporadic dieting and occasionally resisting that second—or third—glass of wine, the tummy bulge has moved in, loves the location, and isn't going anywhere. Good God, Dan, my husband, thinks it's sexy. It makes me feel tubby and old. Add to my expanding waistline is what I call, "noun droppage"—the charming inability to remember names of presidents, books, movies, and countries. Who *was* the president after Gerald Ford? Ford? He was a president, *wasn't* he?

Like my chubby belly, noun droppage, and now this thing on my neck that has a shape and size, a location, and a hard feel under my fingertips, I'll have to learn to live with it. Still, I am not comatose and—a couple of months after first noticing the lump—I mention it to my gynecologist.

"I have a thing, like a knot, on the side of my neck."

"What?"

"I have a lump. It might be getting bigger."

Without a glance, he waves his hand. "You're just fighting a virus, or something. Don't worry about it."

Granted, necks are not his area of expertise, but I accept—am even relieved at—his latex-glove brush off and continue to ignore the little nuisance. With my hair down—the way I always wear it—the lump is hardly visible.

A year later, in September 2005, other symptoms—that I can no longer ignore—indicate that something is very wrong.

Like shortness of breath.

On a recent Sunday, Dan and I begin a two-mile walk. I've hiked the slight but steady uphill trail dozens of times with little effort. But after less than twenty minutes, gasping for breath, I have to stop. Not just to rest, I've already done that twice, but to turn around and go home. This is like Pavarotti pushing himself away from the table without finishing his *Primi* course. It just doesn't happen. I rationalize that my fatigue is because of the pesky little virus, "diagnosed" by my gynecologist, or menopause (boy is that a catchall!), or a funky biorhythm day.

Beside the inability to breathe with any activity, I have night sweats. That symptom gets handily dumped into the menopause bucket. I attribute agonizing leg and foot cramps to too much exertion (which is ridiculous, since I can't exercise).

On the morning of September 15, 2005, I wake in damp, tangled sheets. Turning to dislodge my leg, a searing pain shoots up my back. I gasp, breathe, then ease my feet onto the carpeted floor. Dan has already left for work. Wincing as I stand, and holding tight to the bannister, I make my way downstairs. In the kitchen, I brew a cappuccino and head to my home office.

Along with the back pain, I type my other oddball symptoms into Google. In a nanosecond, the results flash onto my computer screen: a kidney infection. A quick trip to the doctor, a bottle of antibiotics, and I'll be fine. I down three aspirin and call to make a same-day appointment.

# Chapter 2 - Like Hailstones on the Sidewalk after a Storm

BEING ON THE RECEIVING END of someone else's schedule makes me irritable. I hate to wait. I'm writing a To-Do List and crossing and uncrossing my ankles when a jolt of pain shoots up my back. I moan. I sit up straight and the paper on the exam table crinkles beneath me. After a knock, Dr. Gould, my internist, enters. Mid-fifties, balding, too heavy, and all business, he nods. I try to smile. I'm not a doctor-goer and can't remember the last time I saw him. Perhaps I should apologize—for being an alarmist, a malingerer, a time thief—for keeping him from the real patients, the ones who are actually sick.

I describe my back pain as severe and say, "It's probably a kidney infection. That's what Google came up with."

He turns toward his computer. I suspect he's rolling his eyes and thinking, "Oh no, not another self-diagnosing patient with a medical degree from the Internet." He glances back at me, eyebrows raised, "Possible."

"I have other symptoms too."

"Such as?"

"Shortness of breath, night sweats, leg cramps."

"I'll order a urinalysis." He walks toward the door. "Take acetaminophen for pain."

He's been so uninterested in my wacky symptoms that I nearly convince myself to stop right there. Still, I say, "I have a lump."

With his hand on the doorknob, he turns and seems to look at me for the first time.

"What?"

I point.

Instructing me to lie back, he pushes around my neck, under my arms, and palpates my stomach. The room is chilly and too bright, but there's no pain at his prodding. His eyes are closed. *Why is he frowning?*

"How long have you had the lump?"

"I don't know. A year?"

"A *year?* You're kidding."

My eyes narrow, my forehead creases. I don't like his tone. I'm defensive and feel as if he's blaming *me* for this thing on my neck.

"I asked another doctor about it. He said I was just fighting a virus."

Dr. Gould shakes his head as if he either doesn't believe me or cannot fathom the stupidity of his fellow practitioner. Perhaps both.

He turns to the exam-room computer and while typing says, "I'm ordering a workup. Labs first, then x-rays."

I sit up. My shoulders slump as I glance at my watch. I'd promised one of my clients, a large medical center, that a draft of their annual research report would be completed today. It cannot wait, and I still need hours to finish it. Sulking, I walk down two flights of stairs to the first-floor lab. I'm breathing hard when I hand my medical card to the receptionist who calls out, "Stat's here."

*I know what a stat is. Why am I an emergency? This is so weird.*

Whisked to the front of the line, vials of blood, then x-rays are taken. Glad that I've been treated so quickly—while at the same time concerned about the rush—I am too short of breath to climb the stairs and ride the elevator back to the third floor. Dr. Gould waves me into his office, indicates a chair, and closes the door.

He powers up his computer. The familiar sound reminds me of my work deadline. He types, then glances at me with knit brows and appears ill himself. Letting out a long breath, I wonder what a kidney infection looks like and why he corralled me in here to pow-wow about such a no-problem problem. Tempted to say, *Was I right?* I decide to let him go first. My back aches. The computer screen lights up his face. He gazes at the screen, turns away from it, then looks back at it frowning.

Turning the monitor my way, he says, "You don't have a kidney infection."

"Oh." I feel foolish for suggesting it. "I must have tweaked my back."

"I don't think so. A tumor may be the source of your pain."

His words are ambient sounds that don't apply to me.

"Sorry?"

"The pain could be from a tumor pressing on your spine."

Outside the window, traffic moves. The San Rafael Mission with its tall pink bell tower, flanked by palm trees, graces the base of our Northern California hills. The mission bells chime noon. I must get home. I have that project to finish. Everything is the same—reliable, even mundane—yet not at all the same. Objects seem to be moving away from me. I shiver. Leaning cautiously forward, I squint at him and then at the computer.

"A tumor," he repeats.

Cold, I push my hands deep into the pockets of my cardigan.

Pointing to the screen he says, "I don't like the look of all those spots."

Besides the buzz of the computer, I hear a thudding, soft yet distinct.

There's a heart, lungs, and stomach, but also filling the screen are bright spots that resemble glistening hailstones scattered on a sidewalk after a storm.

"Likely lymphoma. I'm sorry."

*Lymphoma? No. No. Cancer happens to other people.*

"Non-Hodgkin's."

"Non?"

"Non-Hodgkin's lymphoma. A type of blood cancer."

"Blood cancer," my voice is disconnected, as if it comes from the walls or the ceiling. I struggle to take a breath.

"Don't worry. It could be easily treatable."

*Don't worry? He said he doesn't like the look of all those spots.*

"I'll call as soon as I have your labs. We'll know more then."

He stands, telling me the visit is over. "You okay to drive?"

I nod. But when I get to my feet, another spasm shoots up my back and I gasp.

"You sure?"

"I'll be fine."

As I walk to my car, I remember that he hadn't ordered a urinalysis. How will he diagnose my kidney infection without a urinalysis? He's not an oncologist. How can he tell me I have cancer? He can't.

I exit the parking garage. In a daze, I slide through a red light and a car honks at me. I wave both of my hands and mouth, "I'm sorry, I'm sorry."

*Jesus, girl, get a grip.*

# Chapter 3 - Hemo Something or Other

I UNLOCK THE FRONT DOOR of our ranch-style house. Spirit, our rescue dog, an aging, overweight, Shiba Inu, and Harriet, our Humane Society cat, a white longhair, lie on our wool entry rug.

When we were told that Spirit was beaten as a puppy, and one of her littermates had been kicked to death, Dan and I had to adopt her. Even though I tempted her daily with table scraps, she spent the first six months after we'd brought her home under our daughter Elspeth's bed, going into the backyard only out of necessity. After a couple of years, she's much more relaxed but still only comes to Dan, and Elspeth, and me. But she does express her love. When I enter the house, she dances around in a small circle. It's light years away from wedging herself under the bed. It's a beautiful dance.

I was more successful at rescuing Spirit than I was at protecting my youngest brother, Johnny, who was also abused as a baby and child. He's gone now—having disappeared when he was eighteen—wanting no connection with our parents, me, or my two other brothers. I can't say I blame him. I tried to shelter him, but perhaps I could have done more.

I close the door and Spirit does her little circle dance. Harriet blinks at me, disinterested, as if I'd come through this door one thousand times before, which, of course, I have. But, actually, no, I haven't. Not this woman with those spots on her x-ray. Not her.

Still cold, I walk into the kitchen and turn on the heater. The pipes clank under the floor. There's a smell of burning dust; it's been months since the heater's been on. I call Dan at his office in San Francisco.

"You sound busy," I say.

"No. What's up?"

"I had an x-ray today that looked funny."

"What do you mean, funny?"

"It had spots, or something." My damp palm grasps the receiver.

"Spots?"

"I don't know. My doctor doesn't either. He said it could be lymphoma, but, of course, he's not an oncologist so how can he know? I think it's a kidney infection."

In the park across the street, sunlight breaks through the leaves of the coastal live oak, creating bright patches on the grass below.

"I'm coming home," Dan says.

"No don't. I'm okay except for this damn back ache."

"But...."

"Stay at work until we get the labs."

"I want to be there."

"All of this may be nothing."

"You sure you don't want me to come home?"

"Yes, I'm sure, and I love you," I say.

In my office—that bright airy room—where I've spent so many hours over so many years, I touch my smooth L-shaped desk. Large black-and-white prints of Paris hang on the wall. Running my fingertips along the frame of a recent family photo—of Dan, Elspeth, and me—I touch the cool glass covering our faces, then turn on the computer.

Waiting for it to come online, I open my month-at-a-glance calendar filled with the scrawl of a busy life: work deadlines, conference calls, yoga classes, dinner parties to host, birthdays to remember. But in this moment of confusion and shock, I feel separated from these activities, as if they describe someone else's life.

I Google Non-Hodgkin's lymphoma, which takes but a bleep to appear: a type of cancer that occurs when a white blood cell becomes abnormal. The cells divide rapidly and will eventually be found in almost any part of the body. Leaning in closer, I read the words again, trying to make sense of them.

I press on my back and flinch. I swallow two more aspirin with the cold coffee on my desk and open the file holding the work project that is due today. I begin to read but can't understand what I've written. I read the paragraph again but keep losing the meaning. All I hear is Dr. Gould saying, "Non-Hodgkin's lymphoma. A type of blood cancer." Blood cancer. My grandmother, Sophie, died of a rare blood disease, in just two days. *Was it Non-Hodgkin's lymphoma? Do blood cancers run in families? My mother called it Hemo-something or other.*

EVEN THOUGH IT WAS DECADES ago—on a perfectly ordinary June morning in 1968—I can still picture my grandmother, sitting at our desk in Los Angeles. She and my grandfather Tom were visiting us. I'd just graduated high school. Sunlight fell onto her smooth arms and bent head. I can visualize her sturdy body, the cotton, floral housedress she wore, and her blue leather wedge slippers. But instead of writing the letter as she had planned, she just stared out the window. I thought it strange but didn't want to disturb her. Tom asked if she was alright. Maybe not. *No.* The doctors admitted my grandma.

The next day, having lost consciousness, Sophie lay in a glass isolation cell in the center of the ICU. Monitors ticked out her pulse, blood pressure, and respiratory rate. In the dimly lit, chilly enclosure, barely large enough for her bed and one chair, I told her I loved her and said that she had to get well. But she did not respond, and I was overcome with a sense of no return. Something had happened that we were helpless to change: *the harsh words you can't take back, remorse about that lover to whom you said goodbye, the doctor shaking his head while looking at his shoes.*

Tom begged Sophie not to leave him. I kissed my grandmother's face, warm but motionless.

In bed that night, I couldn't sleep; all I could see was my grandmother lying in that glass cell. The phone rang before dawn. My mother, Beverly, ran down the hallway into the kitchen and answered after the second ring. At age sixty-eight, Sophie had died, in just two days, from a rare blood disease. "Hemo something or other," is what Beverly called it.

*Did my grandmother have a lump she'd not told anyone about? Was she short of breath? Have night sweats?*

*Do I have Hemo something or other?*

I PICK UP THE PHONE AFTER one ring. It's Dr. Gould.

"I don't know how to say this any differently. Your blood counts are so low you could have a heart attack any minute. You must be transfused. Get to the hospital, now. Right now."

"I'll call my husband. He's in the city."

"There's no time. I'll phone him and explain. Take a cab or call a friend. You must come now."

I call my friend Laurie.

"I need a transfusion. Can you take me to the hospital? It may be lymphoma, but it's probably just a kidney infection. They want me there now."

Packing an overnight bag, I check twice for my sleeping pills, earplugs, sleep mask, and make-up. Laurie knocks and enters in a rush. We hug. Her hair is damp from the shower and she smells of freesia. Seeing her, I feel relief tinged with a vague terror. Relief that I am no longer alone with this bizarre and alarming message from my doctor, but also a sense of terror because she is here to take me away from my home and into a hospital where my life will change in ways I cannot anticipate, into a place where I may lose myself. I dread the prospect of losing control.

Laurie is an attractive woman, three years younger than I, with fine, olive skin and brown eyes. She has a sharply intelligent face and often stands on her toes in photographs to appear taller. Her weight never varies from 108 pounds. During our twenty-year friendship, we have shared much laughter and made many happy memories; but throughout, we have both subtly struggled for the upper hand. There is a whiff of competition between us. I envy Laurie's complexion, her lack of Catholic guilt, and her house with an open floor plan. Laurie might envy my apparent confidence or my career. I don't know.

The hospital is an easy drive through our clean, well-tended city of forty thousand where the climate is Mediterranean. People are polite. We have good restaurants, bookstores, and theaters. Pines, palms, and deciduous trees line the boulevards. San Rafael, twenty miles north of San Francisco, is a lovely place to live.

Laurie passes the Flat Iron Bar.

"Maybe we could stop for a quick drink. Just one."

She shakes her head. "Are you crazy?"

"Maybe a little. But it was a joke. Sort of."

# Chapter 4 - At Home I'd Be Lighting Candles

I SIGN ADMISSION PAPERWORK but don't recognize my signature. An aging, African American orderly in blue hospital scrubs waits with a wheelchair. I'm irritated, not at him but at this whole insane situation. I refuse the seat he offers.

Laurie and I follow him through the colorless hallways where phones ring quietly and people move with purpose across the gleaming linoleum. The wheelchair is empty except for my bright red canvas tote. Over the ambient hospital noise, I can make out the orderly softly whistling, *"Fly Me to the Moon."* We follow him into a private room, number 522, with its narrow bed, fluorescent lighting, and tiny, antiseptically infused, bathroom. The room is warm, and the heater makes a low, whooshing sound while pumping air out of the register.

A faded cotton hospital gown—the iconic garment of all who are sick—lies folded across the end of the bed. When the orderly leaves, I ask, "Do I have to wear that?"

Laurie says, "I'll help."

After removing my clothes except my underwear, I reluctantly put on the gown that she ties in the back. I feel vulnerable and weak, changed from the woman I am—who tries to be kind; who has good taste, or thinks she does; who doesn't eat meat; who reads a lot; drinks a little too much; and wishes she weren't so ambivalent about sex; that woman with those attributes and many more—into a medical record number, lab values, a diagnosis, and a course of treatment. The gown is not who I am. It has nothing to do with me. In just minutes, the hospital has already begun to steal my identity.

After I settle into the bed, the heavy door swings wide; its metal handle strikes the wall like a hammer. Dan steps into the room, then stops. Tall and lanky, flirtatious flight attendants tell him he looks like William Hurt, which he does. With his thick brown hair, combed back from his forehead, he's never had a bad hair day and likely never will. I buy his clothes, and he appears every bit the prosperous, middle-aged executive. I wonder though if the gray suit is too close to the color of his eyes. He looks washed out. Perhaps it is panic. Maybe I look the same.

Dan glances at me, then at Laurie. Jaw set, his forehead is creased with worry and confusion.

"Honey," I say, patting the bed. My voice catches in my throat.

He places his briefcase on the floor and comes to me in two long strides. He puts his arms around me and shudders, as if he's trying not to cry. Afraid that his distress might overtake me, I close my eyes and force down a surge of emotion.

"I'll be fine." I say, rubbing his shoulder.

*What did Dr. Gould tell him? I am afraid to ask.*

He kisses the side of my face, then stands and hugs Laurie, thanking her.

Outside the window, the horizon is crimson; a bat darts in a jagged pattern across the sky; lights cast yellow moon shapes on the walkways. I've seen this all before, but no, never exactly like this before.

Laurie gives us a wan smile. "I'll let you have some time."

She blows me a kiss and leaves with a promise to call in the morning.

Dan sits and takes my hand. "How's the back pain?"

"Better."

"I thought lymphoma was in the blood. Why do you have a backache?"

"It could be a tumor ... pressing on my spine."

"Oh. Jesus."

"It's probably just a kidney infection."

Dr. Gould knocks and walks in. I hope he's not heard me harping about the kidney infection. I wonder again what he told Dan when he phoned him.

After pleasantries, he asks, "May I?" and rubs his hands together.

With eyes closed, he palpates around my neck and collarbones. Then his fingers stop.

"What?" I ask.

"Another lymph node."

"Meaning?" Dan asks.

"We'll know more tomorrow."

"How long am I going to be here?" I ask.

"A day or two. We need to determine what's going on. There's a lab tech outside waiting to draw blood so you can be typed for transfusions. Don't worry. We'll take care of you."

Glancing at Dan, I roll my eyes. Dr. Gould opens the door and the tech enters. She draws the blood sample and leaves.

"I feel itchy in this bed. I want to either get on with it or go home."

At home I'd be lighting candles on the dining room table and pouring myself a glass of Sauvignon Blanc.

# Chapter 5 - Where's My Father Now?

THERE IS A QUIET KNOCK ON the door and a handsome, young Hispanic man enters carrying my dinner.

I thank him as he sets the tray before me.

"How do I get to the cafeteria?" Dan asks.

"Chow hall's on the first floor, but it's closed now."

"Are there any vending machines?"

"Nope. Sorry. But I got another one of these," he motions to the tray.

"You sure?"

"Yeah. There's always extras."

Even though it's past seven and I haven't eaten since breakfast, I grimace as I lift the round plastic cover off the dinner plate. The spinach smells acrid and overcooked, its dark green choppiness giving it away as previously frozen. A shriveled, oyster-colored chicken breast sits atop a dollop of dry white rice. A dish of melted orange sherbet and a carton of low-fat milk complete the meal.

"You might not be so glad you asked," I say.

In a minute, the fellow is back with Dan's tray.

"Thanks, man," Dan says.

"You're welcome. Good luck with that." He motions to the tray and smiles.

The food service gentleman knows about what he speaks. I saw into the muscular meat and jab a piece onto my fork. The desiccated chicken requires sustained chewing, and its excess saltiness puckers my mouth. I look at Dan who is also doing his best to molar the meat into something that can be swallowed. He glances at me and we begin furiously chewing, exaggerate swallowing, then laugh with hands over our mouths. I laugh so hard I'm afraid I might snort the chicken up my nose. But suddenly a pain shoots through my back and the frenetic chewing isn't so funny. "Oh," I say, surprised by the pain. I put down the fork and close my eyes.

"What happened?" Dan asks.

"A back spasm. I'm better now."

He removes both trays to a table, sits on the bed, and holds me.

After a quiet knock, a young nurse walks in pushing a metal "tree" ahead of her. A unit of blood and a bag of saline swing from its horizontal branches. She inserts an IV into my left hand and opens the clamps. The drops fall down the tubing and disappear into my body.

When she's gone, I whisper to Dan, "Thank you, for everything."

"I haven't done anything."

"You have, and you will."

"Of course, I will." He squeezes my hand.

"I'm so tired," I say.

"I know, but we need to decide—about Elspeth. She'll be so upset if we don't tell her."

At the mention of our daughter's name, I feel a shiver of panic.

"What can she do? With midterms. What do we even say?"

"We don't tell her?"

"I don't mean that. Can we please discuss it tomorrow?"

I sigh and clench my hands. Dan looks at me with concern.

"I need the bathroom. What do we do with this?" I point to the tree.

"I'll help."

Dan unplugs the monitor and carefully maneuvers the tree around the bed so as not to pull the IV out of my hand. I sit up and hold my shiny companion for balance while I walk into the bathroom. But its wide metal feet will not allow the door to close. To sit on the toilet, I must pull the tubes as far as possible into the bathroom without yanking them out of my hand.

"God, this is ridiculous." I pee with my left hand extended toward the door.

Washing my hands requires skill and flexibility, as does getting back into bed. The pillows must be just so, the hospital gown not bunched up or open in the back, the tubes and the tree in the precise correct position.

"I hope I can get to the bathroom when you're gone."

Dan gives me a sad smile.

Once I am resettled, I ask, "Did I ever tell you how I almost drowned?"

"No. Where did that come from?"

"This,"—I hold up my hand—"reminds me of it. I couldn't move then either."

"Tell me."

"I was five or six."

"You were still in Wisconsin, before you moved to L.A.?"

"Yes. It was July, maybe August. We'd just come from Mass, and my mother was pestering my dad to drive us to Lake Michigan. He didn't want to go, but she kept at him. He was in a suit; she was in a dress and heels. The humidity was awful. We didn't have an umbrella but my dad laid a plaid car blanket over the sand. I couldn't see the shore on the other side. The sky and the water were just one huge colorless thing."

"Sounds ominous," says Dan.

"It was so hot. I took off my Sunday shoes and socks and walked into the water that ran up my calves. There was a breeze—that smelled of fish and gasoline—but cooled me down. Did you like the smell of gas as a kid?"

"Yeah, I did. Weird, huh?"

"I liked the smell too. So, I stepped in farther and the water felt good. It was still only up to my knees, barely touching the hem of my dress."

Dan fixes his eyes on me.

"Then a speedboat raced by, and a wave broke against my thighs. The next one came quickly and knocked me off my feet, pushed my face to the bottom, and filled my mouth with water and sand. I tried to call out but couldn't make any sound. I couldn't lift my head or get my hands or knees beneath me. It was like being tied down. Like this."

I look at my left hand.

"You must have been so scared."

"Not so much scared as mad that the water kept dragging me forwards then back. My chest began to ache."

"Jesus. How long did that last?"

"Ten seconds? Twenty? I can't say. Then I felt a sharp pressure under my belly. My father yanked me from the water and folded me over his arm. He carried me up the beach then dropped me onto the sand near my mother. I choked and shook. Water ran down my throat and out my nose."

"Were your parents freaked?"

"I don't know. My mother said something like, 'You've got to be more careful.' My dad growled, 'Jesus, look at my suit. It's all wet now.' He still had his shoes on. A lit cigarette hung from his lips. The sun and the smoke made him squint and look really angry."

"I'm sorry," Dan says.

"It was my fault."

"You know that's not true."

"It was to a five-year-old," I say.

"Honey, that's so messed up."

"I haven't thought about that day in a long time."

I look again at my hand tethered to the tree and the bags of liquids falling into me.

"I'm glad you told me."

"Water over the dam. I guess. Or something like that."

"I love you," Dan says.

"I love you too. I'm just so tired."

"I'll stay until you fall asleep."

Dan kisses me and turns out the bedside light. I close my eyes and sink into feeling deeply sorry for myself. I hate that I'm a captive in this hospital room, this bed, and that someone else is controlling me. I yearn for my real life—the busy, beautiful, stressful, ordinary one—that I hadn't appreciated until it was stolen away.

But sleep does not come, except to Dan. For a while, I listen to his regular breathing then softly call his name.

"You should go now."

He wakes and nods his head. "Yeah. I'll see you in the morning."

"I love you," I say.

"I love you too."

At the sound of the door closing behind him, I push down a sob. I gaze around the shadowy room, where windows do not open; where I must do what others tell me to do; where I am tethered to tubes, bags of liquids, and a tree.

Where's my father now to pull me out of this murky prison? Dead, that's where he is.

# Chapter 6 - What Does a *Bunch* Mean?

MY ROOM IS A RESTLESS TIDE: people in, people out, everyone is so busy, swirling around. Even the monitor is busy. Pulse, pulse, pulse. More units of blood and bottles of saline are hung. I always have to pee and jockey the tree and the tubes to the bathroom. Back in bed, my teeth clamp shut. Sleep is impossible.

Sometime after midnight, I can't bear the ruckus anymore and swallow one of my contraband sleeping pills. I doze until a nurse gently shakes my shoulder. It's early; the light in the room is dim and pallid. My head aches. I always get a headache from lack of sleep. The nurse hands me a plastic glass. "Drink this, honey."

"Okay. What it is?"

"Contrast medium. Your prep for a CT scan. Like an x-ray. It doesn't hurt."

"Thank you." I gag down the chalky liquid.

The nurse detaches the plastic tubes running into my IV—freeing me from the tree—and an orderly wheels me to the elevator. We descend alone to the bottom floor where there are no windows in the isolated, underground hallway, just the waxy yellow glow of the florescent lights. He leaves me sitting in a parked wheelchair in front of the CT Scanner Room. I am cranky and impatient but figure that the scan will at least prove that Dr. Gould misdiagnosed me.

*How long is this going to take?*

I'm terrible at waiting. And with blood and saline dripping into me all night, added to the hefty glass of contrast medium I've just swallowed, I slosh with fluids. Bloated and spongy, I worry that with the smallest amount of pressure, I'll start oozing from all sorts of places.

*Can't they please get on with it?*

Annoyed about not having had time to wash up, I run my tongue over my teeth, each feeling as if it's wearing a damp angora sweater. After only fourteen hours as an inpatient, I've become a nondescript, bloated, middle-aged woman wrapped in a flannel blanket, waiting in a hospital corridor with nothing to do except think about when I will get to a bathroom. I've never had a CT scan and don't know what to expect. I had an MRI once and remember having to lie perfectly still. Likely this is the same. It will be hard to relax with a bladder ready to give way.

At last, a skinny tech, who looks alarmingly young, opens the door. *When did he get this job? When he was twelve?* He wheels me inside.

"Back in a minute," he promises, flashing a toothy grin.

Resenting my status as *persona non-grata*, I miss my laptop, my cappuccino, and my mascara. The question won't leave me: *Do I have Hemo something or other?*

I wait. The young tech and his sidekick are laughing and chatting it up behind a glass partition. I want to wave my arms and yell out, "Remember me?" *God, what are they doing in there?* Finally, the boy-tech finishes his happy palaver and comes at me with a large hypodermic. I flinch.

"No worries. This goes right into your IV. We're just gonna top off that contrast juice."

*Oh God, not more fluids.*

Lying flat, he glides me into the narrow white tube and leaves the room.

"Okay. Don't move," he says over the speaker system.

The CT scanner whirrs, clicks, and clanks. My arms are at my sides. No fight or flight. All I can move are my eyes. The beams of the scanner penetrate my body and produce an image of my insides that emerges onto a computer screen in the next room.

"Hold your breath," he says over the speaker system. Then a few seconds later, "Okay, breathe."

*Click. Whirr.* The sounds remind me of the idle of a taxi—the unfamiliar clatter that woke me one morning when I was nine years old. I walked from my bedroom to the open front door of our Los Angeles home where a man picked up two of the three suitcases at my mother's feet.

*"Mama?"*

*Dressed in a black coat, high heels, and a small blue hat, she startled at my voice and turned toward me. I didn't move, just watched her, and felt the warmth of sleep and my bed drain away. The man picked up the last bag. No one else was awake.*

*"Does Daddy know?"*

*She nodded. Her face looked old in a way I'd not seen before. She stepped forward and put her arms around me, then let go. Without looking back, she turned and closed the door. Her high heels tapped across the driveway. All that was left was a hint of her Shalimar perfume.*

*I shivered. My legs were weak, and I reached for the doorknob to steady myself. After the noise of the taxi faded away, there was quiet. Holding the knob until the light became more yellow than gray, until the heater came on and warmed me, until there was nothing else to do, I walked into my parent's bedroom.*

*"Daddy," I said, shaking him by the shoulder.*

*He didn't move.*

*"Daddy," I said, louder. He opened one eye. "You gotta get up now."*

Click. Whir.

"Don't breathe. Breathe." The tech's voice comes over the loudspeaker and startles me out of my reverie.

More than anything, I want to bolt. What world is this? Tap, tap. *Let me out. That's what my mother did. She got out. She was gone a long time.*

Finally, the tech announces. "That's it. You're done."

He slides me out of the scanner

"Thank you," I say, always striving to be kind.

*"No problemo."*

Anger flares in me.

*What a stupid thing to say. Why in the hell would I be here if there was no problemo?*

"Okey, dokey," he chirps as he wheels me into the hallway. "Somebody will be right here to wheel you and this chariot back to your room."

I sigh. The door closes and there I sit again, only now the urge to pee is critical. Crossing my legs tightly, I look up and down the hallway for a bathroom. Nothing. I'm too self-conscious to knock on the CT door and ask the boy-man for assistance with my desperate, middle-aged bladder. The *no problemo* comment makes me angry all over again. I know it's a generational thing; so many young people don't know how to say you're welcome. It bugs me whenever the no problem comment is thrown my way, but today it is especially galling. Then Dan strides around the corner. Thank God. Relaying my immediate crisis, he rushes me back to 522 where I toss off the blanket and dash to the bathroom. Then I brush my teeth, floss, then brush again.

Breakfast has arrived: doughy, undercooked pancakes, orange juice that likely started out as powder, incinerated sausages, and coffee, so weak that I can see the bottom of the cup. Why can't the coffee be as black as the sausages? I have a serious Jones for a French roast cappuccino, hot and strong, something I brew at home every morning with my espresso machine. I sip the watery, lukewarm coffee. Awful. You might think that after a cancer diagnosis and being warned of an imminent heart attack—all in the course of one afternoon—that anemic coffee, inedible food, or a lack of privacy wouldn't matter. Well, they do. To me.

Dan sits facing me on the bed. Gesturing toward the tray, I ask, "You want this?"

He shakes his head and looks me straight in the eyes, "I told Elspeth."

I frown, upset that I hadn't been involved in telling her. But then I feel grateful and relieved that the terrible chore is over. My shoulders and face soften. Elspeth and I are so close that Dan must have hated to break such shocking news.

"Last night I drove part way home, then pulled over and phoned her. I had to."

"Did you mention cancer?"

"Only as a possibility." He glances at his watch. "She's finished her exams and is coming home."

I want to know how Elspeth reacted but am too physically and emotionally depleted to ask. Dan looks as exhausted as I feel.

"Thank you," I whisper.

I can't ask if he cried, or if Elspeth did. I hope that—despite the awful message—it was a conversation in which they felt closer than ever. More vulnerable, yet stronger; kept afloat by that tough, sometimes tatty, little life raft that is family.

"Is she okay?"

Dan nods. "I also called your brother Randy."

"How is he?"

"Upset. He wants to talk to you and thinks you should call Beverly."

I hadn't thought about telling my mother. What would I say? That I'm in the hospital, getting transfusions and tests, for what, they don't exactly know? Beverly is seventy-eight and not in great health; is it even fair to burden her with this piecemeal information? Is it kinder to keep it from her? Given our fractured relationship, I wonder how much she would even care.

"Randy wants to be there when you tell her."

Randy was the golden boy. The Paul Newman look-alike. Athletic. Good in school. Popular. Beverly's favorite.

"He's such a better person than I am."

"Honey, that's not true. But he thinks Beverly might need help dealing with this."

"Whatever *this* is," I say.

After the dismal breakfast tray is removed untouched, a tall, handsome, and lightly bearded doctor—who could have made good money as a regular on General Hospital—enters my room. The two black earpieces of his stethoscope peer out from his lab coat pocket like the eyes of a baby marsupial. As a hospitalist—a doctor who cares for people while they are inpatients—he has the dubious good fortune of giving me the outcome of the CT scan. He introduces himself as Dr. Arent.

"I have your results," he says thumbing through papers before rolling them into a tube that he grips in both hands. I glance at Dan, smile, and give him a thumb's up.

Dr. Arent begins by assuring us that the dose of radiation I'd received—less than 60 mGy—is harmless. Whatever an mGy is. He continues to spout clinical jargon such as computed tomography, axial, and sagittal planes. Whatever they are. Geometry was never my strong suit. I'm beginning to tune him out; his voice is becoming a buzz. Then, in the middle of one sentence about ionic contrast medium, he mumbles, "A bunch of lymph nodes showed up."

Glancing at Dan, I shake my head as if to ask, "Did you hear that? Did you get it?"

"Excuse me," I interrupt, "but what does a *bunch* mean?"

Is this another medical term whose definition is essentially different from that in common usage? He looks at his hands, now grasping the paperwork so hard that it collapses into itself. Then he describes the lymphoma as "multi-site," "extensive involvement," "stage 4."

*Oh. What?*

With a great deal of sympathy, he says, "I'm sorry. I am really, really sorry."

Dan has the same stricken expression as yesterday. He reaches for and squeezes my hand. Dr. Arent sits down on the bed and I smell soap, nothing flowery, more like mint or thyme. He puts his hand on and then strokes my right calf, which lies outside the sheet. I regret that I hadn't shaved my legs in a couple of days. Through the tears, the stubble troubles me. I try to come up with an intelligent question about the scan but keep thinking that on my deathbed I'll want my legs to be smooth. My vanity is also stage 4.

His words are so unexpected, so contrary to how I feel that they strike me as crazy. Perhaps I could have understood, or accepted them, had I been in terrible pain. But I'm not. The backache has subsided. All I want is a damned cappuccino. A person who is so desperately sick isn't thinking about coffee.

*He cannot be talking about me, about my body.*

"Ask the nurses if you need anything." He lets go of my leg and stands. "And remember, if you're gonna get cancer, lymphoma is a good one to choose."

He is so kind and wants to help me feel better. He smiles and walks out of the room.

"I can't believe it." I shudder in Dan's arms. We cry, then cry some more. Finally, we inhale deep, trembling breaths and release each other. I wipe my runny nose.

"My God. He cannot be talking about me." I sniff.

Dan wipes his eyes with a crisp white handkerchief.

"I don't understand," he says. "How can lymphoma just happen?"

*How can it?*

I feel a twinge of guilt and point to my neck. "Maybe I should have paid more attention to this."

"What is it?" He squints.

"A lump."

He leans toward me. "Yeah, I see it."

"I've had it a while."

He waits for me to continue.

"A few months, maybe more. I thought it was a virus. That's what one doctor said."

I cover the lump with my hand.

"Why didn't you say something?"

"I don't know. I believed it would just go away."

"I get that, especially if your doctor told you it was only a virus," Dan says.

"I trusted him when he said it was nothing. I wanted to believe it was nothing."

I turn away from my husband. Outside the hospital window there is only haze. The world is uncertain, indistinct. I don't know this place. Neither of us do.

My shoulders drop. I turn back to Dan. "I'm so afraid."

He reaches for my hand. "Me too."

# Chapter 7 - "Hola Mamacita"

ELSPETH OPENS THE DOOR and takes just one step into my room. She's never seen me sick. Not like this sick. She glances at the unit of blood, bottle of saline, the tubes inserted into my IV, and the flashing monitor. I must suppress an urge to cry out, to say, "It's me. It's really me. I'm here."

"*Hola Mamacita*," she says, smiling while disbelief and dread flicker across her face.

"*Hola, Hija*," I reply, using our familiar greeting.

A blonde, self-confident wisp of a thing, Elspeth's smile is dazzling, the result of years of orthodontia, an expected practice in childhood these days. Her clothes might appear too casual, a bit reckless, but no, the peach tones in her jacket piping are the same as those on the vintage handbag slung over her shoulder. Her ivory-colored shoes, which could be dismissed as inconsequential, are likely couture. The jeans that hug her exceptionally long lean legs, the same. All carefully foraged from one of the many L.A. second-hand designer stores she haunts.

Her steady gaze is filled with love and devotion. This is the moment my daughter changed. The moment that mortality became not just a concept, or something that happened to very old people, but a clear picture: her own, fifty-five-year-old mother lying in a hospital bed being kept alive with pints of blood. I ache that she has to see me like this.

Elspeth walks in, sits on the bed, and buries herself into me.

We hug for a long time but neither of us cries. Crying would be an admission, and nothing is as yet certain. I nestle my face in her neck that smells like honeydew. Not having washed my hair, I hope it is not stale. Finally, we unwind.

Elspeth embraces Dan. They look at each other like people who share a bitter secret: *the dog must be put down, you didn't make the team, the groom hasn't shown up.*

Elspeth sits back on the edge of my bed.

"You look beautiful," I say.

"You…."

"I look like hell. My legs are a stubble factory and my face is totally puffed."

I bring my hair closer around my neck. Elspeth has never noticed the lump either, but, of course, she lives in L.A. and has her own life.

"*Mom,* how are you?"

"I'm okay. Just tired. This place is a madhouse at night."

"Sounds like student housing."

We both laugh. Dan does too.

"I'm glad you're here. But I wish you didn't have to be."

"I get it, Mom. Me too."

"Tell me about school."

"Tell me about *you.*"

"Nothing much more to say. Yet."

"Mom?" She looks me straight in the eyes, her voice challenging me for more.

*Now who's withholding information? What did Dan tell her? Why didn't I ask him what he said and what Dr. Gould had said?*

"Anything new since last night?"

I glance at Dan and give my head an infinitesimal shake.

"I don't think a kidney infection has been completely ruled out, but if it's cancer, the doctor said that lymphoma is a good one to choose. Right, Honey?"

"Right," Dan says, but his response is more of a question than an answer. He is so honest that he gets bollixed up with white lies; and I can see his discomfort knowing at any moment he could blurt out more than I want him to.

"Very treatable is how my doctor described it yesterday."

"Oh Mom." Elspeth rubs my hand.

After a soft knock, my friend Tina, with her long, dark hair and yellow silk scarf, slides into the room. "Thanks for coming, Sweetie," I say, my voice wavering. She kisses the side of my face.

"Laurie called me. Wild horses and all that," she says.

Tina and I have known each other since we were both pregnant with our daughters. We became friends right away. She's intelligent, warm, and has her own artsy-spiritual take on everything. She writes, and sculpts, loves an ice-cold martini, and a game of poker. Laurie, Tina, and I, along with our husbands, have played penny poker for years. Relieved that she is here, I think there will now be space between Elspeth and me; and, for the moment, I will not be forced to answer her simple question: *How are you?*

Dan perches on the wide windowsill. Tina and Elspeth sit on chairs next to my bed and begin discussing Ang Lee's new movie, *Brokeback Mountain*. Dazed, Dan watches them, his forehead creased, as if he is trying to comprehend, but his eyes are unfocussed. He is clearly not present.

Is he thinking I could die? I could almost accept the idea of Dan's remarrying—someday, far in the future—but the idea of Elspeth having another mother makes me livid. No, I can't stand the thought. *F-it.* I am her mother. We share everything. Who did she tell when she had her first sexual experience? Me, of course.

*We were in my car and had just pulled into our garage. Elspeth finished the revelation with, "Mom, it was over so fast."*

*I laughed out loud and said, "You go girl."*

Maybe not the most appropriate response from the mother of a sixteen-year-old, but there it was. Relief spread over her face.

When she was six and I caught her in a lie, we stood together in the kitchen and she sobbed in my arms, telling me again and again how sorry she was. Perhaps she felt that she had broken something that could not be fixed.

But I told her that I loved her, more than ever for wanting so much to be honest with me. In the coming years, I bought her prom dresses, tampons, tickets to the Backstreet Boys. We danced together in the aisles at *Rent* and *Mama Mia*. I am determined that I will be with my daughter in the dressing room grimacing at the price tag on her wedding dress.

*I will not be replaced. I am not dying. I will be the only mother Elspeth will ever have.*

This conviction is built of love and a fierce protective impulse. There is no border where the love for my daughter ends.

It has been an enduring pain in my life that my mother did not have those same powerful instincts toward my brother, Johnny. Beverly's love for her youngest son never began, but her disdain for him had no limits. *Why?* Hers was a grim story and maybe it's not up to me to judge her or my father. I'm not going to go into extended detail about growing up in a household with a raging, alcoholic father and a narcissistic mother who became addicted to pain meds. It's just too sad, too pointless, and we've heard it before. But I will relay the bigger picture that reveals why Johnny disappeared and what he ended up doing with his life.

# Chapter 8 - The Biggest Mistake of Her Life

BEVERLY DESCRIBED HER LIFE as a string of bitter disappointments. She'd had her heart set on attending the elite and private Northwestern University at Evanston, Illinois; and she would have gotten in, except that in 1945 the GIs were coming home and they got first-admission priority. Fair enough, but Beverly felt herself too good to attend the University of Wisconsin at Madison, where she had been accepted.

Then, in defiance of not getting into N.U., she made the dopey decision to live at home and work at her father's neighborhood grocery store, certainly not a magnet for eligible bachelors. Four years later—and still working with her dad—all of her friends had married and, at twenty-two, she thought of herself as an old maid. Then a friend arranged a blind date with her and John Shultz, a handsome navy vet and student at U. of W. Thinking him fresh, Beverly slapped his face on their first date.

Believing she could do better, she didn't want to see him again. While a college man, John came from struggling farm folk. Beverly's family was doing well in the grocery business and she considered herself socially superior. But John wouldn't give up and she agreed to see him again, and then again. His first proposal came within a few months. She accepted, then after wedding invitations had been mailed, she changed her mind and broke it off. But he wouldn't take no for an answer.

Beverly was afraid that she would be a spinster and work forever in her dad's grocery, which was just too awful. John seemed to be her only other choice and he eventually convinced her to marry him—again—a move that she would describe repeatedly as the biggest mistake of her life.

Eight years into a petulant marriage, they had me, Tom, and Randy.

Dad was restless and determined to get out of Racine, a city too small for his ambitions and the persistent gossip about his drinking. But it was Beverly's hometown. All her friends and family were there. She deeply objected to the move, but John got a job transfer to California, and she went with him.

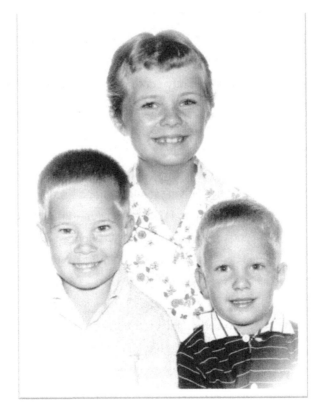

*Susie 8, Tom 6, Randy, 4*

In Los Angeles, they fought all the time, and she was going to have another baby.

In May 1957, their fourth child, and third son, was born. They brought him home from the hospital without a name. We called him "Baby." When the hospital social worker telephoned, needing his name for their records, I pressed the receiver against my belly and shouted to my mother barricaded in her bedroom.

"The hospital needs a name for Baby."

"I don't care."

"What should I tell them?"

"Call him Johnny."

This baby would be named after his father, perhaps to placate John, perhaps to remind and punish him. It hardly mattered.

To keep him out of her way, Mom tied Johnny by the wrist into his crib. She used a green cotton, cord-like belt from a summer dress she no longer wore.

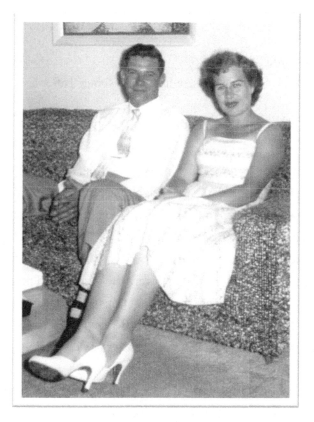

*John and Beverly*

On a hot, airless summer morning, Dad leaned over Johnny's crib with a kitchen carving knife and yelled, "You will never, never tie this child up again."

Mom stood, shaking with fury, behind him. "You have no idea what I go through."

My father sliced up the green cotton belt. Beverly didn't try to take the knife away. I was as terrified of the knife as of my father's rage.

"You are an unfit mother," he roared, hurling a piece of the sliced-up belt at her.

Johnny wailed from his crib. Wide-eyed, Tom and Randy whimpered as we witnessed this trauma in the boys' shared bedroom.

"I hate you," she yelled.

"Shut up," Dad screamed.

"Go to hell."

"I'll report you."

Dad stormed out of the house while Mom shouted after him, "You son of a bitch."

I began to lift Johnny from his crib, but she shoved me aside. "Out. All of you."

Then she pushed us three older kids out the front door and locked it. Tom and Randy followed me into the hot, bright glare of the street. We walked up a neighborhood hill that led to the highway. We needed shade and something to do. I was so thirsty. I was so scared.

Without a traffic light, a crosswalk, or a median, Tom, Randy, and I— like under-sized sprinters—leaned in toward the four lanes. The heat made the cars speeding toward us from both directions look far away and wavy. Glancing left and right down the highway, I thought the break in the traffic would give us enough time.

"Okay."

Yanking Randy's hand hard, the three of us darted across the super-heated asphalt. At only four years old, Randy's little legs could barely keep up. A car honked, then another. The boys panted, their faces were red and splotchy. The blazing sunlight made them squint. I licked my upper lip and tasted salt. My heart pounded. Standing at the side of the highway, the hot asphalt smelled like singed coffee.

"Let's go this way," I said, trying to pull Randy down a narrow street with no sidewalks. He refused to move. "Maybe there's a park down here."

"No. I wanna go home."

"We can't. We're locked out."

His hand slipped out of my damp grasp. He threw himself onto his belly and pounded the dry, weedy dirt with his fists. The toes of his scuffed shoes slammed into the ground as he continued to rant.

"Get up," I yelled.

He howled. Tom, unable to say or do anything, stared at Randy. I needed to stop his tantrum. Sometimes he would get so mad, he'd stop breathing.

"Okay. Quit bawling," I cried. "We'll go back."

I pulled Randy to his feet. We waited a long time for an opening in the stream of cars before we dashed back across the highway.

My head throbbed as I turned the knob and the front door opened. I glared at our mother, sitting on the living room couch, smoking a cigarette.

"You shouldn't tie Johnny up."

"You don't know anything," she yelled.

Johnny was still in his crib crying, not tied in but behind a closed door. I lifted him out. After that day, I always took him out of his crib.


DAD LEFT ME AND MY brothers alone in public places. Mostly it was parks, but sometimes it was stores or burger joints that were so far from home we didn't know where we were. With his jaw continually clenched and his knuckles white from his grip on the steering wheel, Dad would pull his car over to the curb and say, "Get out." He'd give me a couple of dollars and disappear.

One time, thrusting bills in my direction, he told Tom, Randy, and me to go into a department store and buy our mother a bra for Christmas, describing numbers and letters that I couldn't understand or remember. Embarrassed and rummaging through boxes of bras, I hoped no one would notice us. But a saleswoman came over and asked what we were doing. I told her. The woman said not to worry about the bra. Waiting for our dad to come back, we wandered around the store. When he finally returned, the woman, looking angry, took him aside. He said something and then she said loudly, "Take your children and go home."

The smell of alcohol and cigarettes was sickening. That's what my father's anger always smelled like and it filled up the car. I looked straight ahead and didn't make a sound. I tried to say, "I'm sorry. I couldn't find the bra," but I was too afraid and the words wouldn't come. I gave him back his money.

He also dragged me into taverns. I hated them and often threw up on the drive home.

It took another year, but Mom finally delivered an ultimatum: your wife and kids, or Gordon's Gin. Dad left us, four shell-shocked children—and never enough money.

Terror of my father and the need for his love created a fission that would burn within me for a lifetime.

## Chapter 9 - "I Love Best the Curly Hair"

"I AM NATALIA GREYZ."

A glamorous young woman—with a stethoscope draped around her neck—holds her hand out to me. I wonder if she's met the handsome Dr. Arent. They would make a striking couple. She wears no doctor's lab coat, just a navy sheath under a salmon-colored wool jacket with her name, Dr. Greyz-Yustapov, pinned on the lapel.

"Everyone calls me either Dr. Greyz, or just Natalia. I have no preference. Yustapov can be difficult."

"Hello, Dr. Greyz." I shake her hand. I will never call her Natalia.

"Good to meet you. I am your oncologist."

*My what? Why did an oncologist just barge in here? I never asked for an oncologist.*

Hyperventilating, I put my hand to my solar plexus trying for a slow, deep belly breath.

Dr. Greyz has impossibly high and rounded cheekbones, green eyes, and thick, wavy, auburn hair. When I look at her, I feel none of the relief I did at seeing Laurie or Dan. Just fear. I pull the thin cotton blanket around my shoulders. I do not believe she will be the bearer of good news; why is she so sunny? Why do I feel like I'm auditioning for Dr. Greyz—who must ask herself the same dreadful question each time she walks into a new patient's room: *Will or won't this patient survive?*

After introductions, Dr. Greyz turns to Elspeth. "So, you are ready for the graduation?"

"Yes, next spring."

"Good for you."

Dr. Greyz looks me in the eyes and I think, *here it comes*. My secret exposed. Elspeth will learn the truth. My jaw tightens.

"I've reviewed your results. Your lymphoma is stage 4. This is called distant spread."

Feeling protective, I want my girl to leave, but she takes my hand. Dan puts his arm around Elspeth's shoulders. They steady and ground each other.

"To get the better picture of your lymphoma, we must perform the biopsy."

Dan mouths, "I'm sorry."

"This will tell if the cancer is in your bone marrow."

I wipe my forehead with the back of my hand.

Dr. Greyz continues. Treatment will likely involve vats (my term) of chemotherapy; I will become sterile (not a problem at fifty-five); and my vital organs might not survive. Dr. Greyz's monologue of side effects makes all of us frown. I try to smile at Elspeth but my mouth trembles and won't obey.

"Your hair, it will fall out," she says.

This strikes me as funny. "Seems that's the least of my worries."

"When it grows back, it becomes the dark and curly type."

"The chemo silver lining. I'll look like Andie McDowell."

Dr. Greyz also seems pleased with this side effect and says, "I love best the curly hair."

With this upbeat remark and Ukrainian syntax, she smiles. "See you soon." She waves and exits the room.

We all look at each other. I burst out laughing. "No kidding? Andie McDowell?"

"Mom, you'll be a new you."


AN HOUR LATER—once again disconnected from my tree—an orderly appears with a wheelchair to collect me for the biopsy. The novelty of the

Andie McDowell hairdo has worn off, and we leave room 522 in a somber pack.

Tina and Elspeth wait in the oncology reception area. Dan accompanies me into the procedure room. Dr. Greyz asks about symptoms and feels around my neck and under my arms, turning to make notes on her computer.

"I don't really like doing this one," she admits, glancing at a small tray covered with a white towel that has "Sterile" printed on it.

I'm not sure if this makes me feel better or worse, but I appreciate her honesty.

*I'll get through this. I will. I'm shaking, but I'm okay.*

Oddly enough, at just twenty, I'd assisted at several of these procedures. Thinking some day of going to medical school, I worked part time in a San Francisco pathology lab where I cooked up microbiology agars, cultured specimens, and assisted with bone marrow biopsies. The patients enduring these tests suffered. One woman clamped onto my hands and screamed for minutes on end. Medieval seemed a good description of boring into bone with a large-gauge needle and sucking out the marrow. The anguish of those patients haunted me. Now I was one of them.

"Please lie on your stomach."

Turning over, I settle onto the rustling paper. Dan reaches for my hand. His is warm in mine that is cold and sweaty. Dr. Greyz opens the back of my hospital gown and asks, "Ready?"

"Yes," I reply. My heart pounds against the table. *What choice do I have?*

After cleaning the site with alcohol—its sharp yet sweet smell reminding me of the times as a child I'd been terrorized by my needle-wielding pediatrician—Dr. Greyz shoots a syringe of lidocaine deep into the back of my right hip. I wince and grip Dan's hand.

"Okay?" she asks.

"Yeah," I mumble into the table, struggling to get a full breath.

After the lidocaine, the placing of the biopsy needle feels more like sharp pressure than the searing heat of the anesthetic.

"I am into the bone."

*Okay, I am getting through this.*

Then a painful vacuum sensation begins. "Your hip is producing a good amount of marrow. This is excellent."

"Great," I murmur.

"Next, I must retrieve a piece of the bone."

Retrieval is intense but short. Dan must have peeked because his eyes appear glazed over; he is pale and looks as if he might faint. Dr. Greyz removes the needle and bandages the biopsy site. Dan helps me into the wheelchair. Wrecked and beat up, I lean forward to avoid putting pressure on my sore hip. Dr. Greyz puts a drop of the bloody marrow from the syringe onto a slide and studies it under her microscope.

"Is there cancer?" I ask.

"It is a good sample."

"Do you see lymphoma?"

"You did very well." She looks at me. "And you too," she says to Dan. She smiles her perfect smile.

"But lymphoma is a good one to choose, isn't it? I mean if you have to choose." My voice is pleading, squeaky. "That's what Dr. Arent said."

"We will have the pathology results in a couple of days and then you will see me again. I would say to stay away from the computer."

*Right.*

Dan wheels me back to the reception area where Elspeth is asleep on Tina's shoulder. My daughter stirs and opens her eyes. Her anxious face makes me want to howl.

I know the seven warning signs of cancer. Do I think they don't apply to me? I am an idiot and blame myself for creating this. This nightmare. After twenty-four hours as an inpatient, I am discharged—ancient, rickety, profoundly apologetic, and ashamed.

*A new me? I don't want to be that woman, no matter how cool her hair is.*

# Chapter 10 - Distant Spread

EARLY THE NEXT MORNING, I brew a cappuccino. Heaven in a porcelain cup. I know stage 4 cancer is the last stop before death, but I've not heard of Distant Spread. I turn on my computer.

*F-ing Google Hell.*

I sip the coffee and re-read the paragraph. To paraphrase: in distant spread malignancies, cancerous cells from lymph nodes spread through the bloodstream to almost any part of the body where they then set up their murderous (my adjective) colonies.

*No.* My body cannot be gorged with cancer cells. This drivel does not apply to me. It pisses me off. My hip is sore from the biopsy, but the intense back pain from two days ago is hardly there. If that pain is caused by a tumor pressing on my spine, how can it be gone now? Somebody's made a whopper of a mistake.

With a second coffee in hand, I stand in my bright, but empty, living room. Weeks ago, Dan and I ordered new furniture and trekked our old stuff down to Elspeth in a U-Haul. As nothing new has yet arrived, our living room contains only one red upholstered armchair and a lot of echoes bouncing off the walls and hardwood floor. With a new deck coming in, we'd also had the backyard dug up. The nearly empty living room and the churned-up, dirt-clod backyard strike me as apt metaphors for my newly overturned, dissipated life. Distant spread is also what happened to our furniture.

Sunlight floods in through our four French doors facing the east San Rafael hills covered in oaks, madrones, and bay laurels. I breathe in, expanding my diaphragm, and out, long and slow. My shoulders drop. My bare feet soak up warmth from the wooden floor. The swaying treetops are jade green, the trunks emerald. Above the ridgeline, a marine blue sky is streaked with clouds the color of pewter. Swallows dart and lift on the thermals. The beauty of the morning is so piercing, it's almost painful.

Opening the doors, I smell foliage, dirt, and the salt ocean just a block away. The scent of living things. Everything is alive, but alive in the way that I am in this moment. Madly conscious. Blood buzzes in my veins; I am not sick but ruthlessly okay. Another deep breath. I smile. What has changed in the world? Did grace, biology, or an alignment of the planets produce this momentary perfection, loss of ego, merging of the self with all that lives outside the body? Is this vision a suit of armor against the terror of cancer, or is it a glimpse into the foyer of death? Or heaven? In any case, it's okay. I am safe. I close my eyes and feel life pulse through my body.

All is well. All will be well.

# Chapter 11 - Everybody's Getting Cancer

SIPPING MY COFFEE, I watch the silver clouds trail across the sky and wonder if Dan and Elspeth will think my joke about distant spread and our furniture is funny.

Randy will call soon. He and his wife, Diane, are driving the one hundred miles from their town north of San Diego to Beverly's home in Los Angeles. They want to be with her when I reveal the lymphoma. As our aging mother spends most of her time in bed, I can picture them—ready with hugs, compassion, and Kleenex—in Beverly's pink and blue floral room with Randy perched next to her on the bed, and Diane sitting on the vanity bench in front of the huge mirror, draperies drawn.

The phone rings. I pick up. It's Randy.

"Here you go," he says and hands our mother the phone.

"Hi Mom," I say, thinking Mom more appropriate than Mother or Beverly for this as-intimate-as-it-gets-between-us conversation.

"Oh, my knees are *really* aching." A long sigh. "You know, I don't think I'm ever going to get any better. Not any better."

"I'm sorry ... I have not-great news too," I say.

"Are *your* knees bad now?"

"No. No. Nothing like that."

"Thank God. I wouldn't wish this on anyone. Not on my worst enemy. Doctor Gilbert says that all I have left is just bone on bone."

"Mom."

"That's why I have so much pain."

"Mom?"

"The pills hardly help at all anymore."

"Can you listen? *Please.*"

"I am listening."

A beat of silence. "I have lymphoma."

Beverly says nothing and I wonder if she's heard me, but then she clicks her tongue, sighs again, and says, "Just about everybody I know is getting cancer."

I can feel the creases tighten across my forehead as I take the cell phone away from my ear and look at it. Beverly goes on.

"Gwen's husband, Mel, he's had lung cancer for years and will not give up. Gwen was sure he was a goner last year. But he's still here."

*What?*

"And then there's Marylou's son…."

Beverly drones on with one dismal story after the next while I reply, "Oh dear," to all of this woe. At last Randy takes the phone.

"Can you get on the extension?" I ask him.

He picks up in the kitchen.

"Beverly, you can hang up now," I say, my voice flat.

The receiver clicks.

"What the Effing hell?"

"I guess I misjudged that one. Sorry, Sis."

"Geez. She sounded as if I'd told her I couldn't get my newspaper delivered on the porch and she's heard the same damned thing from everyone else."

"You didn't deserve that."

"Why did I even bother? If it's not about her, it's not important. And you drove a hundred miles to be with her for this useless phone call."

Deep breath in; blow it out.

"Did you get any more information yesterday?"

"No." I lie to protect him, to protect myself. "The doctor said that if you're going to get cancer, lymphoma is a good one to choose."

We hang up and I whisper, "Lymphoma is a good one to choose."

IF IT'S POSSIBLE TO CHOOSE an illness, Beverly chose hepatitis and arthritis. To be fair, she had been hospitalized for hepatitis after Randy was born. She recovered but after her divorce she suffered regular bouts of chronic hepatitis that put her securely into bed for weeks at a time. The hepatitis struck whenever she overdid it, which happened a lot. She was raising four kids on her own: we were fed, the house was clean, bills got paid. I have to give her credit for all of that and when it became too much, perhaps she isolated herself with illness. It seemed she needed a break during which she could do little, or nothing at all.

She had regular bouts of hepatitis until, in her sixties, osteoarthritis became her main squeeze. During a particularly serious flare-up, I—then married and in my thirties—flew to L.A. and drove my mother to a doctor's appointment.

*"So, Beverly," her doctor asked, "can you describe the intensity of pain you're experiencing?"*

*I expected to hear adjectives like excruciating, unbearable, and unrelenting, instead she said, "I don't really have much pain—but I'm afraid I might."*

I was dumbfounded. Speechless. The agony that had laid my mother up in bed for over a decade didn't *bother* her? Is it possible to be incapacitated by *anticipation* of pain?

On another occasion, I visited her in L.A. during a bad "spell." Beverly had gotten her doctor to write a prescription for a high-dose, transdermal Fentanyl pain patch. As the dutiful daughter, I hurried to the pharmacy and had the prescription filled. Back at her home, I ripped the patch from its multiple layers of hard-fused plastic and offered it to my mother.

"You know. I don't really need that now. Maybe I might tomorrow."

Really? *Really?*

"I'll just take a Vicodin."

Ah, yes, Vicodin. Narcotics shed a bright light onto Beverly's bizarre relationship with illness. While she wasn't actually experiencing pain, she believed that agony could strike at any moment. Better pop a precautionary Vicodin. I figured she'd been stoned for years and loved that floating sense of inertia that allowed her to do little or nothing during her career years as an invalid.

*Why?* That was another issue. If pressed for an answer, I would say that my mother didn't deal well with disappointment, still harbored rage against my father, and had become addicted in the process; and the narcotics created a reality for her that was impenetrable to others. Drugs and hypochondria provided a hard shell against the world and gave Beverly ironclad control over what she claimed she could and could not do.

"I'm not up for that," became my mother's mantra.

Beverly's exit from everyday life made me determined to do the opposite. My impression of my mother: she was weak, even stupid, for lying around in bed wasting her life. Because she was also angry and even cruel, especially to me and to Johnny, I had little sympathy for her. Beverly had chosen her destiny as invalid and I would do everything I could to never become my mother.

# Chapter 12 - Tijuana Tonic

ALL DAY THE DOORBELL RINGS, and I forget about my mother's bizarre and flat-footed comments. Friends and neighbors bring bread, soup, pie, casseroles, and humorous books like *Cancer-Schmancer*. The diagnosis comes up now and again, but no one dwells on it. We sit together for a few hours during a warm, luminous September afternoon. Dan brings dining room chairs into the empty living room, we drink mineral water, and pass around bowls of salted cashews. If I weren't sick, I'd be far too busy for this afternoon of just sitting around. I'd have a To-Do List of a dozen items.

While it's only been two days since my diagnosis, I've already missed a deadline. I emailed my client to apologize but was vague in my reason for Nondelivery of their project. I assured them I'd finish it in a few days but seriously wondered if I'd be able to fulfill my promise.

Late in the afternoon a neighbor, Monica, dressed in a turquoise velour running suit, comes by. Her patchouli oil takes me back to my hippie days. Monica leans over and whispers, "How much have they told you?"

"They?"

"Your doctors. Are they being honest with you?"

I remember Dr. Greyz studying my marrow under the microscope and not answering my question about the presence of lymphoma and Dr. Arent dismissing my CT scan as a "bunch" of lymph nodes. How would he have left that conversation had I not asked for the definition of a *bunch*?

"We're still waiting on test results," I say.

"You gotta be the squeaky wheel. Otherwise, they won't tell you a damn thing."

"I'm not afraid to speak up."

"Good for you. What are you going to do?"

"What do you mean?"

"Are you just going to let them pump you full of poisons? I'm only saying this to help you think about your options."

"My oncologist,"—the term sounds all wrong and when I say it, I feel as if I have a ball of tin foil in my mouth—"said a lot of chemo will be involved."

"Chemo isn't the only way."

"You mean alternative medicine?"

"Yeah." Monica's long beaded earrings jostle against the sides of her face. "It's worked for so many people."

"Like who?"

"Like Kris Carr."

"Who?"

"Kris Carr. She's amazing. She calls herself a healing junkie and is super famous. She was diagnosed with stage 4 of some rare and horrible cancer that was all over her liver and lungs."

Monica sweeps her hand through her short, hennaed hair.

"But instead of bombarding her with toxins, her doctors decided to just watch and wait."

"No radiation? No chemo?"

"Nada."

"Wait a minute. She had tumors polka-dotting her lungs and liver, and her oncologists did *nothing?"*

*"Nothing."*

"Well, that's some big-ass magic," I say, in need of a bit of levity.

Monica shakes her head. "I don't think so. Kris *believes* that health and illness are two sides of the same coin. She writes about seeing her tumors as beauty marks."

"What?"

"Sounds crazy, I know, but it worked for her. It could work for you. I'm just saying."

"I don't know if we can just do nothing."

"If it were me, I'd at least consider alternatives before frying my cells."

"Hmm. I … don't…." I stare at the top of my left hand where there is still a mark from the IV.

"I'm sorry. I didn't mean to upset you. I'm just passionate about helping," Monica says.

"It's fine. You didn't upset me. It's all so new. But I will ask about the watch and wait thing."

"You know, I have a friend who was diagnosed with lymphoma."

"Oh?" I lean towards her.

"She did a lot of research on alternative treatment and located a clinic in Tijuana."

The mention of Tijuana makes me suspicious. *Not exactly the Mayo Clinic, is it?*

"They do cutting-edge work in micronutrients and vitamins."

"Is she cured?"

"Not really."

"What happened?"

"Unfortunately," Monica shakes her head, "she passed."

"Oh."

"The treatment didn't fail. She just hadn't started the micro-nutrients soon enough. They told her that, before she died."

The micro-nutrient-Tijuana-treatment thing makes me cringe. I would have to be in the most desperate, end-of-the-line, situation before traveling to Mexico to try and save my life with micro anything. I "get" Western Medicine. Its view of the body as an essentially cause and effect universe with a strong chemical and mechanical response makes sense to me. And oncologic pharmaceuticals have a direct and dramatic effect on quickly dividing cancer cells. Intellectually, I can get behind this straightforward, measurable approach. I've never been an "alternative-medicine" type, and I'm not about to start chugalugging micro-nutrients any time soon. If I have to go down the treatment rabbit hole, I'll take my first swig from a bottle of chemo. Emotionally, though, the thought of chemo makes my teeth ache and my center clench.

"Listen, I gotta go, but tomorrow I'll send you all the clinic information," says Monica.

Which she did. I laughed out loud at her email. What else was there to do? But I hesitated for just a moment before I deleted it.

# Chapter 13 - Mom's To-Do List

DAN, ELSPETH, AND I ARE HAVING brunch at the Half-Day Café in Larkspur, an upscale college town ten minutes from our home. My veggie omelet appalls me. The sheen of oil on it is so distasteful that all I can do is push the eggs around my plate with a fork. Elspeth and Dan glance at my mutilated *huevos*. It's only been three days since the diagnosis, but, in that time, so much is different. I've seen the sky tremble with color, as if it had a pulse, a heartbeat. Sound moves through my body. I might cry at any moment. And food is almost intolerable. But deep in this maelstrom, this ever-shifting kaleidoscope, there is an occasional sweet ripple of acceptance and perfect calm. In those moments, I breathe easy and my muscles relax, become soft. There is quiet. Time stops.

From our café table, I gaze out the window at our local Mt. Tamalpais. Over the years, I'd organized many outings to the Mountain Play—an annual musical theater extravaganza. It draws thousands of people who sit on stone seats for hours in an amphitheater on the top of the mountain that's often baking in the full sun. (When it is particularly hot, attractive young men run up and down through the crowd spraying lucky people with water guns.)

I'd pack an elaborate picnic for the six or eight friends in our group. We'd spend the afternoon eating, drinking, and watching the play. Afterwards, several of us would walk the seven miles down the mountain to our cars. Then, we'd all congregate back at our house where I cooked and served a three- or four-course dinner. I'd put everyone up for the night and prepare breakfast in the morning. Today, I wonder if I'll ever be able to accomplish that iron-woman triathlon of entertaining again.

"Hey Mom. How you doin'?" Elspeth brings me back to our table.

"Good. Thanks," I say, trying to sound cheerful and present.

"It's cool to be at the Half Day with my Parental Unit."

I smile at her familiar Parental Unit endearment.

Thinking it might make all of us feel as if life hadn't been whacked completely out of recognition, I'd suggested Sunday brunch at the noisy, cheery café. People laugh and wave at friends across the room, kids roam in curious packs from table to table, and fry cooks yell out orders from the open kitchen. But the ambient din makes talking difficult unless you're good at conversing next to a power mower. Gazing at all these gregarious, athletic people in spandex bike shorts and visors makes me feel fragile and lacking. I reside in a separate world and looking normal is the most I can hope for. In seventy-two hours, this cancer has already isolated me from their world of activity, a world in which I just recently thrived.

"You know what the nurses call Dr. Greyz?" Elspeth asks.

I shake my head. "No."

"The Double-Oh-Seven Girl."

"Really?"

"I get it," says Elspeth. "She sure is hot and has a lot going on upstairs."

I laugh at the nickname for my stunning Ukrainian doctor, okay, *oncologist*.

After breakfast, we drive to Blackie's Pasture, a wide spot in the road named for a beloved horse and the site of a popular trailhead that leads to the exclusive seaside village of Tiburon. It's another limpid, late-summer afternoon. Even Spirit seems excited. She jumps onto the back seat from the floor, sticks her nose out the window, and sniffs.

We take a short stroll to a bench overlooking the San Francisco Bay. Spirit trots along beside Dan but avoids me. Is it my imagination or is Spirit more standoffish than usual? Can she smell the cancer? Does it frighten her?

I ask Dan, "Can you take a picture of me before I lose my hair?"

Dan snaps photos of me alone and me with Elspeth; we even nudge Spirit into the frame. Sunglasses obscure my face. I've lost more weight and appear thin, diminished.

"Let me get a picture of you and Dad," I say.

Dan and Elspeth sit on a bench, the dazzling bay behind them. She is in front of him, with her knee bent and her left foot flat on the bench. She'd forgotten her tennis shoes and is wearing a pair of mine, which are prominent in the frame. I take the picture with my cell phone and as I look at the image, I imagine myself gone, as if my shoes are all that's left. The picture terrifies me.

"Let's take a walk," she says.

Too fatigued, I decline. Elspeth, Dan, and Spirit take off down the shoreline trail. Sitting cross-legged on a flat rock near the lapping water, I breathe in the briny smell of the ocean. The lethargic, green waves of the North Bay flow up onto the dun-colored sand then make an equally drowsy return to the sea. Pelicans, with their primordial profiles, glide silently across the cloudless blue sky; while gulls, craving attention—sort of the Buster Keaton of birds—squawk and perform clown-like acrobatics.

Watching the tide, I search for that quiet place within, the one I felt yesterday morning when I gazed at our hillside. But I can't reach it and begin to brood. This lymphoma has already sliced and diced my psyche into different characters: I am the stubborn woman, hand on the wheel, determined not to lose control; the solitary little girl panicked by what the doctors have in store; the idiot denier profoundly apologetic for, and embarrassed by, my oblivion; the psychedelic tripster reveling in a world of color, sound, and emotion so intense I can hardly bear it. Had I been alone on this beach, I might have cried or ranted. Instead, I breathe and accept that the only thing to do is to take my splintered self back to the hospital tomorrow for more blood transfusions.

Dan, Elspeth, and Spirit come rushing up the path.

"We gotta go. She's gonna miss her plane," Dan calls.

Before this illness, I would have been eagle-eyeing the time; but today, deep in my despair and isolation, time and airline schedules have no meaning.

We hurry to the car—as quickly as I can hurry. In the back with Spirit, my dog moves to the other side of the seat. Delayed by heavy traffic, we arrive at the Oakland Airport just forty minutes before Elspeth's return flight to Los Angeles. There's no time for long goodbyes, for which I am both grateful and terribly sad. I dread Elspeth's leaving and taking her loving, comedic self away.

"You've got to call me all the time and let me know everything," she says.

"I promise."

"I'll be back soon. I love you."

"I love you too," I say.

Then she runs toward the terminal, her cheap Costco carry-on bag flip-flops behind her. I wave and blow my daughter a kiss, but she's already turned a corner.

Back home, I lie down, exhausted. On my bedside table, she's left a note.

*Mom's To-Do List This Week:*

*1. Creative Visualization*

*2. Think Positive*

*3. Call Elspeth all the time and anytime*

*4. Take the best care of self*

*5. Cry*

*6. Laugh*

*7. Shave legs*

I press the paper to my chest, then smile. Elspeth has given me a list of what to do. I so need guidance of any kind. In a fetal position, I hold my fractured self together. Closing my eyes, I am profoundly grateful for how well my daughter is helping me prepare for what lies ahead. Whatever that may be.

But there is also the strangeness of my daughter taking care of me. Of my daughter being in my role, of wearing my shoes, so to speak. I might have to get over that, at least for a while.

## Chapter 14 - A Cancerous Mush

THE NEXT DAY, I am back in room 522 again and around my bed are a tangle of tubes, monitors, and flashing numbers. Saline, units of packed cells, and pints of platelets have been pumped into my veins for hours. Exhausted, my only exercise is padding back and forth to the bathroom.

I didn't expect to see Dr. Greyz. She enters my room and walks to the edge of the bed.

"These,"—she points to the plastic bags hanging from the tree—"will make you feel better."

"That's what I hear."

My smile is wan; so is hers.

Dr. Greyz looks out the window. I follow her gaze. It's late September. The days are getting shorter. I wonder, *How can I be here?* I don't belong inside this hushed, smoke-colored building with linoleum floors and fluorescent lighting; where I am little more than a collection of dreadful lab values and test results; where people wear latex gloves to touch me and often hold something with which to pierce my body. Dr. Greyz turns back to me.

"This I hate to tell you. The biopsy showed lymphoma in your bone marrow."

Her hands rest on the blanket. I try again for a deep belly breath.

"With cancer in the marrow, it can't produce the good healthy blood cells. Your red and white cells and your platelets, are at the low, low levels. I am sorry to report this."

Reaching for my ChapStick—anything that is real—I open the tube and push it around my dry lips.

"How much? Do you know how much lymphoma?"

"About ninety-eight percent."

*What?* I don't know whether to laugh, or cry, or tell her to stop with the bad jokes.

"Are you saying that ninety-eight percent of my bone marrow is cancerous?"

Dr. Greyz nods. "These things are hard to hear."

"Are you sure?"

"Yes."

When she looked into her microscope after the bone marrow biopsy, all she saw was cancer. She must have been afraid for me but she's a pro and her expression revealed none of that fear.

*Has she ever looked at a slide of bone marrow and seen nothing but cancer?*

"A heart attack is still a problem. So is bleeding."

*How is it possible I'm still alive?*

"I'll be careful with razors." I can't think of anything else to say, and I sound pathetic, even to myself.

"A cut is not the problem. A platelet count as low as yours could result in a brain hemorrhage."

I cannot believe that Dr. Greyz is talking about me. *My bone marrow. My heart. My brain.*

"How could this have happened?"

"Your question is a good one. The causes of lymphoma are mostly unknown. Why a patient has this…?" She shakes her head and shrugs.

What is a shrug—an acceptance, a giving up, a rolling over? Rubbing my damp palms on the bedspread, I wonder if I am ready to give up.

"Next, we must learn what type of lymphoma you have. The pathologist will make a report from the biopsy slides before we can say for one hundred percent."

"Will it matter?"

"Yes."

"In my treatment and…?"

"Everything."

"Dr. Arent said that lymphoma is a good cancer to choose."

Dr. Greyz smiles and gives her head the slightest nod.

"Do you agree?"

"You will come to my office on Friday. We will have the better picture then."

"I don't know what to say."

"Questions will come up. Bring them with you."

I swallow. Fear tastes like salt. Why didn't Dr. Greyz answer my question about lymphoma being a good cancer to choose? I twist the cap of the ChapStick.

"I know I have revealed a great deal but try to not worry." She squeezes my hand. "I'll see you Friday."

I doubt it. I'm already missing. I don't even have marrow, just a cancerous mush that multiplies inside my bones and is trying to kill me.

# Chapter 15 - You'll Be Gone by Halloween

ON FRIDAY, DAN, ELSPETH, and I sit in the oncology waiting room for the diagnostic appointment with Dr. Greyz. I mull the possibilities. Greyz—*grays*: to make ashen, to grow old, to die. Or *graze*: to feed, devour, decimate. I'm on a trajectory. As a child, my pediatrician's name was Dr. Kruel who'd terrified me with his needles and polio vaccines.

I count the empty seats—twelve—and wonder if that is a good sign, or not. We huddle together on a narrow beige sofa. Dan taps his right foot against the gray-and-black-flecked carpet. Elspeth—who flew up from L.A. and insisted on being with us for this important meeting—holds both of my clenched hands in hers. I smell my daughter's toothpaste or Altoids.

The reception area looks like a Courtyard Marriott. Its prodigious neutrality numbs the senses and blunts the emotions. *Is this intentional?* What effect would the room have if the walls sported photos of all those who had beaten the odds—smiling cancer survivors with clean CT-PET scans and robust bone marrows? Tossing frisbees to golden retrievers, taking that second honeymoon to Cabo San Lucas, or roasting marshmallows with grandkids in an idyllic campground. Even in an oncology waiting room— maybe especially in an oncology waiting room—ambience matters. A spot of yellow would be lovely here.

A sturdy, middle-aged nurse shows us into the same exam room where I underwent the bone marrow biopsy. Glaring early-autumn sunlight streams in through long windows. No rainfall all summer has singed the hills into barren mounds where last spring's grasses, lupine, and California poppies had thrived. Elspeth and I perch on the tissue-papered exam table; its rustling sends acid into my stomach. Dan stands to my side, his hand rests on my shoulder. Dr. Greyz walks in wearing a white lab coat over pleated brown slacks and a pair of obviously expensive tan-and-brown flats. More beautiful than ever, the 007 Girl's skin is flawless while I, with an increasingly puffed-up face and persistently clammy palms and fingers, am becoming more frog-like every day. The doctor is so young; she could be my daughter. I search her face for some clue of what is to come.

She shakes my damp hand. Hers is warm and dry.

"Well," Dr. Greyz begins. I tell myself to pay attention. I would love to let my mind wander, to be spared the message this morning.

"Based on the pathology of your bone marrow biopsy, we understand you to have Mantle Cell Lymphoma." Her lips purse as her forehead creases. "I was ninety-nine percent sure of this Mantle Cell when I viewed your marrow under the microscope; but the pathology report is a necessary confirmation."

Even though Dr. Greyz holds nothing with which to pierce me, I feel as vulnerable as I had during the biopsy. I realize that she's known, or strongly suspected, the type of cancer I have as soon as she looked at the slide of my bone marrow (or the cancerous mush masquerading as my bone marrow) in the exam room. Distrust begins to creep in but I can't afford that; I need an ally. I need her on my side. My left eye begins to twitch. I hate it when that happens. It's always from stress and makes me feel stupid and out of control.

"Mantle Cell Lymphoma is a rare cancer. It is both aggressive and indolent at the same time—"

Dan interrupts, "Can you please explain that?"

"Yes. Aggressive lymphomas grow quickly, and are life threatening, but respond better to treatment than indolent lymphomas, which are slow growing but harder to destroy."

Her words run together. I'm having trouble concentrating, but the message is clear: *the worst of two worlds.*

"MCL, excuse me, Mantle Cell Lymphoma, is like both. It grows and spreads quickly and is difficult to eradicate for any length of time."

Dr. Greyz glances at Elspeth, then at me, her eyes saying, *I'm sorry.*

Like the pull of a breaker at the back of the legs as it rushes out to sea, I feel my life being sucked away. My hands tighten around Elspeth's, as if to hold on against the retreating tide.

Dr. Greyz pauses then studies the wall over my head. "But we have some things working in our favor. That you are fifty-five years instead of sixty-five or seventy is a plus. And your heart and lungs are strong. They can take the chemo."

"And what is the chemo?" I ask, my voice wispy.

Dr. Greyz reviews Hyper-CVAD (Cyclophosphamide, Vincristine, Adriamycin, and Dexamethasone), the big guns she'll fire at the MCL. The aim of this chemotherapy cocktail (regimen is her term) is to bombard the cancer with as many chemicals as possible—in the shortest amount of time—wiping out the lymphoma before killing the patient. (She doesn't mention killing the patient, but that is the subtext.) Hyper-CVAD is given in two courses, A and B, with the mixture of drugs differing in each. The maximum number of courses any patient can tolerate is eight, four of A and four of B.

After she finishes, as if to let this sink in, there is silence. I stare at the computer screen as if looking for answers. I turn toward my daughter whose eyes are closed.

Then I ask, "You mentioned what I have working in my favor. What isn't working?"

"Stage 4 with bone marrow involvement. These are not working."

Even though I'd asked the question, I am annoyed with Dr. Greyz for answering it. I want to send Elspeth out of the room. Of course, she wouldn't go.

Dan asks, "Will she get the chemo here, in your office?"

"No. Due to side effects, the Hyper-CVAD can only be given in the hospital." She looks down at her stylish shoes and shifts her weight.

I want Dan to thank Dr. Greyz for her time and tell her that we won't be needing her any longer. I want him to usher us out of this room and back into the life I knew just a few days ago. We should go out for lunch, somewhere nice. Maybe Tiburon or Sausalito, a place with a view of the Bay.

Dan asked, "Should Elspeth finish school or come home?"

*What a good question*, I think. If I could choose, I'd be selfish and want Elspeth here where her affection and humor would lift my spirits and ease my pain; but interrupting or postponing our daughter's graduation seems like a needless, even extravagant, move. As a mother, I want my daughter's life to be as unaffected as possible; as a cancer patient, I want her here with me.

"I would vote to stay in school," replies Dr. Greyz. "You have what, only some months for graduation? Right?"

"Yes. Eight," Elspeth replies.

"And L.A. is not so far."

She'd remembered where Elspeth went to school. She does have a lot going on upstairs. Another beat of silence. The annoying question thrums in my head. I feel melodramatic asking it; still, I blurt out, "What are my chances?"

"We haven't cured the MCL." Dr. Greyz clasps her hands in front of her.

Dan squeezes my shoulders. Elspeth leans her head against mine. Confused, I wonder, *Am I giving up or just beginning to fight? What am I supposed to say? Or do?*

"But a long-term remission is possible."

"Long term?" Dan asks.

"Median survival, after diagnosis, is about three years. After four years, survival rates decline, but *why*, that is unknown."

The light coming in the window is too bright and I shift my eyes away.

"But don't forget, median means that half of the people live *longer* than three years."

Elspeth breaks the surreal mood by piping up, "Mom, you are not a statistic."

"That's right," Dr. Greyz agrees, nodding her head. "You are not a statistic."

I smile, but think, *Why aren't I a statistic?* Half of Mantle Cell patients go through chemo and are dead in less than three years. Fifty percent live somewhat longer. Not a statistic? Actually, aren't I either one hundred percent alive or one hundred percent dead in three years? Isn't that the only statistic that matters? What can possibly get me into some elite MCL club where my outcome will be vastly better than anyone else's faced with this dreadful disease? Nothing makes sense.

"Have you ever heard of Kris Carr?" I ask.

"No," Dr. Greyz shakes her head.

"What if we just watch and wait? See if I need chemo after all?"

She looks me straight in the face. "You will be gone before Halloween."

Halloween is five weeks away. I glance at Dan. He looks at me as if I am a long way off, and I realize that I am. No wonder he is confused and might think of me as if I am someone else. I am. I've become a sick person. I've never been really sick and have no practice. What does a sick person say, or think, or do? Do they make plans? Do they rail against their illness or accept it quietly? Certainly, some pray, but that's not my style. I hardly know where to look but glance at Elspeth who gives me a tired smile while tears fall down her face. I stand to indicate that I am done with this conference.

"Thank you, Dr. Greyz. I don't know what else to say."

"Call my office when questions come up. Don't rely on the Google."

"Okay." There is no way will I be staying away from the computer.

She smiles. "Don't worry. Our Hyper-CVAD ammunition, it will do the jobs."

"Yes." I nod.

We are silent as we leave the office and walk down the linoleum corridor. The slight squeak of our footsteps makes me want to run. Dan, holding my hand, presses the elevator button repeatedly. The pleasant, helpful ding signals the arrival of our escape route, but as we step into the hospital lift, I feel as though I am entering a silo, a place where I will be separated from everything I've chosen, built, and thought I controlled. I will be placed in a room where the windows won't open, where the grayness is oppressive, where the lighted numbers on monitors will replace candles, linen napkins, and black-and-white photos of Paris. I take my first step into the new world of Mantle Cell Lymphoma and am already changed forever.

# Chapter 16 - No Long-Term Survivors

*COME ON.* DID DR. GREYZ really think I wouldn't Google Mantle Cell Lymphoma?

Except for the hiss of the coffee machine, the house is quiet; it's Saturday, and Dan and Elspeth are sleeping in. I put both hands around the heavy, blue porcelain cup and sip the hot bitter coffee. A taste of home. I relax my shoulders. While my computer beeps to life, I look around my office.

The French doors let light into this space where I disappear but not in the way I disappear into the hospital. It's the opposite. I'm at my most focused, productive, and competent in this room. I look forward to coming into my office every day to feel creative and helpful. My career is not over. I am not done here. There is much more to do.

The three photographs of Paris that hang over my desk were taken on an early Christmas morning—the same day and time that Dan, Elspeth, and I arrived there a couple of years ago. Tree branches are bare. The foggy sky looks cold. The pavement is wet. A lone bird sits on the back of a park bench. Dan doesn't like the pictures. Too somber he says, too bleak, but I tell him they remind me of our *merveilleux* trip to Paris.

I don't know why people complain about the French; I find them delightful. Flirtatious waiters, people who stop on the street to help you find Notre Dame, wine less expensive than bottled water, and how delicious it is to say, *Bon Jour, Bonsoir,* and *Merci Beaucoup.*

Everything was fine our first night in Paris. Coming in from the cold drizzle, the warm little cafe felt like an embrace, a kiss on each cheek. The ceiling was strung with tiny white lights. A dozen or so diners sat at iron-and-marble bistro tables. Laughter, the clatter of heavy dinner plates, and the chef calling out orders for pickup—his words sounding like poetry—were the perfect soundtrack for a holiday dinner in France. The small menu was written on a chalk board: meat, fish, or chicken. The short, sturdy tumblers at the ready for red or white house wine by the carafe.

We were buzzed, carefree, and celebratory. A young girl, wearing a pink sweater and a purple tutu, romped around making friends with everyone. She did a perfect plié when I told her how lovely she was in her tulle and ribbons. A well-dressed older woman sat alone at a table nearby. Everyone, the little girl too, was French but spoke good English to us, the obvious Americans. I wondered why these people weren't home with families. What were their stories? We spoke with the older woman, as did the little girl, and I wanted to ask her to join us but felt too self-conscious. Now, I wish I had. What was there to lose? Regret is sour.

Our trip to Paris was almost two years before my diagnosis. It's likely that cancer cells were already reproducing in my body but hadn't yet formed a palpable lump. I'd never heard of Mantle Cell Lymphoma. Who knew cells had mantles, or capes, or cloaks? Cloak in French is *manteaux*.


MY FINGERS TAP THE FLAT, black keyboard making a confident, even energetic sound—life moving on as if nothing is wrong. With a confirmed diagnosis—or a seemingly confirmed diagnosis—I square my shoulders before reading.

*Mantle Cell Lymphoma is one of the rarest of the non-Hodgkin's lymphomas ... the outlook for those with advanced or recurrent disease is poor ... MCL is considered incurable.... The clinical outcome of MCL is dismal, with a median survival time of 3 years and virtually no long-term survivors.*

Incurable. Dismal. Three years. No long-term survivors. So much for Dr. Arent saying that lymphoma is a good cancer to choose. Perhaps he's never heard of the rare Mantle Cell.

I return to the kitchen and brew another coffee. While the dire statistics hold a morbid curiosity for me, I cannot accept that the abbreviated life spans of MCL patients will be my fate. Even with cancer having elbowed out my bone marrow, I am confident I will get well. I will not die. I don't know how or why I know this. I just know it. *In my bones.*

I wonder if Elspeth or Dan will Google MCL. Of course, they will. Everyone will.

I can't read any more studies and instead look for cheap flights to Paris.

# Chapter 17 - "I Can Torture You"

IT'S MONDAY. ELSPETH FLEW back to L.A. yesterday. Dan and I wait in the drab, hotel-chain décor of the Ear, Nose, and Throat reception area, the same interior as in Oncology. But here the mood is casual, even nonchalant. A visit to ENT might mean nothing more than touchy tonsils, swimmer's ear, or an annoying postnasal drip.

A nurse shows me and Dan to an exam room where I will have my neck sliced open to remove the lymph node that will be a secondary confirmation (or not) of the bone marrow diagnosis of Mantle Cell Lymphoma.

Dr. Downing, a blonde, pert, no-nonsense woman in her forties, enters. "Sorry," she says, "but there's been a mix-up and my anesthesia assistant didn't show. I can torture you and take the node out myself with a local pain killer, or we can wait."

"As much as I want the ugly thing out of me, I'm not going to opt for torture," I say.

"That's probably wise because before you can start chemo, you will need a VAP implanted into your chest, which will require a second surgery anyway."

"A what?" Dan asks.

"A VAP. A Venous Access Port."

"What's that?" I sound defensive and argumentative even to myself.

"The VAP is the point of entry for the chemo which will then bypass any delicate tissues of your arms or hands where it could be irritating." She rubs the top of her left hand.

"So, you're saying that this VAP thing is going to be put into my body?"

"Yes. The idea behind the VAP is that your veins will be spared and won't collapse with repeated sticks."

"How's that?"

"You'll be stuck in the chest instead of the arm or hand."

My shoulders slump.

"If we remove the node at the same time the VAP is inserted, you'll be under a general anesthesia."

"I can choose oblivion over suffering?" My tone is decidedly sarcastic.

"Yes." Dr. Downing nods.

The node excision is rescheduled for two days later.

"What the hell," I say as Dan drives us home.

"I'm sorry, Honey. That was a surprise."

"What else do they have up their sleeves that we don't know about?"

At home I pay bills and am struck by the ghastly reasonable question: *Will I expire before my VISA card does?*

# Chapter 18 - Deep Sympathy for My Newly Assembled Self

ONCE AGAIN, I LIE IN 522 and wonder how this room is always available to me. Having just been wheeled up from recovery, my persona as cancer patient is complete: the VAP—the chemo superhighway—has been implanted into my chest and the malignant node has been removed from my neck. My body now belongs to my doctors, my insurance company, and the pharmaceutical industry. And no one is wasting any time.

Dr. Greyz sweeps through the door. "I am happy to say we start the Hyper-CVAD tonight."

She is effervescent.

"How long will Susan be here?" Dan asks.

"Eleven days, maybe twelve."

"What?" I say. "How long?"

Dr. Greyz is a kind person, but every time I see her, I feel as if I've been mugged.

"We must quickly wipe out as many cancer cells as possible."

I sigh.

"Honey, we need to be tough," says Dan, my chemo promoter.

"Yes," agrees Dr. Greyz. "But I know you can handle this." She smiles and encircles my hands in hers.

"Do you have any questions?"

We shake our heads and Dr. Greyz leaves 522.

Woozy from the general, I close my eyes and place my fingertips on the flat bandage on the side of my neck. For the first time in a year, I can't feel the hardened node, the knot. It's been leveled like a condemned building, spent like a child's tantrum, disgorged like a bad seed. The malicious thing that I had successfully ignored, that my gynecologist had dismissed as a pesky virus, that thing is gone.

Hearing someone enter the room, I open my eyes. A nurse holds two bulging bags of clear liquids. This is the moment. This is how it starts. I am not afraid. I am not glad. I am resigned. Like when I was in labor, 8 cm dilated, and they wouldn't give me any more pain meds. Point of no return. The only option was to push. Birth that baby. And that's what I did. That's me again, now. No turning back. Push ahead. Take what comes.

I can feel the weight of those bags and their coolness, sense how the liquid sloshes inside the heavy plastic. The liquid makes me aware of how thirsty I am. I ask Dan for a glass of water. The nurse hangs the bags on the metal tree at my bedside. Then she wipes a spot under my left collarbone with alcohol, pushes a needle into my chest, and connects the chemo tubes. A monitor for exact dosing begins its quiet, regular beeping, measuring the drops that might return me to my spectacularly average life.

Dan and I watch the clear chemicals seep down the tubes into the VAP in my chest. I listen but can't hear anything; the plastic tubing swallows the sounds of the drops falling. I wait for a feeling, a warmth in my chest, a stinging in the veins. But there is nothing. No smell. No sound. Just a flutter of hope.

# Chapter 19 - Expiring of Fatal Constipation

*"BY THE SEA, BY THE SEA, by the beautiful sea,"* is the cheery tune my cell phone plays and wakes me every morning at home. Today, I open my eyes to the clicking of the room heater. Still dark outside, the red numbers on the chemo monitor blink and bleep their all-okay. Steady as she goes.

*"You and I, you and I,*

*Oh, how happy we'll be."*

The coffee is again weak and terrible, but the aftereffects of the general anesthesia have given me a good night's sleep. I am ready to take whatever son-of-a-gun pharmaceutical warfare they have planned for me. I will sail through chemo in record time and be cured.

*"When each wave comes a rolling in,*

*We will duck or swim...."*

The first full day of Hyper-CVAD has me lashed to the bed like Gulliver. Numerous tubes connect my VAP and IV to no fewer than five bags of fluids that hang from the metal tree. While the chemo drips into my VAP, units of blood, anti-nausea drugs, saline, and bicarbonate drip into the IV in my hand. With all this fluid flowing into me around the clock, my major activity is shuffling back and forth to the bathroom. Saturated from the mid-section on down, my legs are becoming waterlogged trunks and my feet are swollen and turgid. Whenever I move (waddle), I swear I hear sloshing. I pee every hour, which leads to another lab value: measurement of the number of cancer cells I urinate, meaning that I can't even flush the toilet. All of my urine goes into a "hat," a pink plastic contraption installed under the toilet seat. Apologetic to the aides who routinely have to pour all of this into a beaker and deliver it to the lab, I offer to do it myself but the nurse's aide says, "Aw, Honey, this ain't nothin.' I see worse all day." What an angel.

I also take oral antibiotics, antifungals, antivirals, stool softeners (that don't do a damn thing), and the lovely tranquilizer Ativan for nausea and anxiety. But as the level of chemo increases in my bloodstream, biliousness becomes a constant companion.

Day four of chemo marks the beginning of the free fall of my white cell count. This expected outcome of treatment means that I will need daily injections of Neupogen to stimulate the production of white blood cells in the bone marrow (if there's any marrow in there).

An oncology nurse shows Dan and me how to inject Neupogen, which we will need to do daily when I am back home. I wonder if Dan can give me a shot. He's never been fond of needles, but he takes to it right away. I, too, become adept at piercing myself in the gut—yet another target area in the endless onslaught of needle sticks.

By day five, the chemo is wiping out normal blood cells right along with their homicidal cancerous cousins. Even with continual transfusions, my red cells, white cells, and platelets remain at "the low, low levels," as Dr. Greyz describes them. Being so kick-ass, Hyper-CVAD must be given in small doses to minimize side effects. I guess that's why this first round is so long.

Besides exhaustion, I'm quite certain I might expire of fatal constipation, a side effect of nearly every med they pump into me and a source of persistent discomfort and exasperation.

Dr. Greyz visits almost every day. I ask her to prescribe a laxative that is "nuclear." She thinks that's funny and orders a double dose of Dulcolax that doesn't help at all.

Here, in hospital room 522, my customary anxiety and impatience for even brief inactivity has been forced to take five. My usual mental clamor has been chemically gagged. My extra critical superego has chemo brain too and hasn't quite found the new vocabulary with which to condemn me and my lethargy.

During the first five days of chemo, I've accomplished almost nothing except emailing my clients to let them know that their projects will be delayed. I haven't wanted to reveal this but have no choice. Saying nothing is worse than the truth. While I don't get into detail, I tell clients I am in the hospital for cancer treatment. Missing deadlines and not meeting obligations is so unlike me, no matter how understandable the excuse. I never want to be looked at as unprofessional and have no intention of giving up even one of my clients, no matter what lies ahead. My clients email back and are all understanding and concerned about me, not their projects. This gives me considerable relief.

But there is more in my life now than cancer, chemo, and missed deadlines; there is also newfound and unexpected joy. There is depth in connection and simplicity. There is beauty in small gesture.

The brilliant Christopher Hitchens, while gravely ill with esophageal cancer from which he eventually died, wrote about friendship. From his memoir, *Hitch-22*:

*"Another element of my memoir—the stupendous importance of love, friendship and solidarity—has been made immensely more vivid to me by recent experience. I can't hope to convey the full effect of the embraces and avowals, but I can perhaps offer a crumb of counsel. If there is anybody known to you who might benefit from a letter or a visit, do not on any account postpone the writing or the making of it. The difference made will almost certainly be more than you have calculated."*

*A CRUMB OF COUNSEL.* I love that. And it is true. My friends understand this and visit, bringing gifts, and laughter, and sentiments of caring. My friend, Jeanne, and her husband arrive one afternoon with a high tea including lemon cake, current scones, cucumber sandwiches, and tea in a thermos. We indulge as if we are being feted in an English manor house. Another evening, they bring an entire Chinese dinner for four. Dan sneaks in a bottle of wine. We feast on the intensely fragrant food. Even without touching the wine, I am giddy in my hospital bed.

If generosity were an Olympic sport, Jeanne would take the gold; and Laurie is always there for me—driving me to appointments, staying with me in the hospital, and calling friends. Others bring books, scented lotions, and homemade breads. Kindness overwhelms me. When friends walk into room 522, my world changes. The beautiful outside comes in. Full, bounteous life enters. Connection brings sunlight into the glacial grayness of cancer.

DAY SIX, I GOOGLE Hyper-CVAD and learn that cyclophosphamide, the C in Hyper-CVAD, is a form of *mustard gas*. And Adriamycin, the A—known as the *red devil* because of its bright crimson color—is so toxic that blistering, ulceration, and persistent pain at the site of injection may require surgery of the damaged tissue followed by skin grafting. This cancer drug is so badass that there is a *lifetime* limit on how much of it people can tolerate. Mantle Cell Lymphoma must be a monster to require this arsenal of toxic drugs.

Then I Google the side effects of Hyper-CVAD, described in the medical literature as *complex and numerous*. Few body parts or systems are spared. One of the hardest hit is the digestive system. You name it—from the mouth on down—and Hyper-CVAD messes with it.

*Nausea and vomiting are common but some anti-nausea drugs can cause constipation.* No shit. Excuse me, but that is an entirely accurate response.

*Hyper-CVAD can cause diarrhea* ... Oh, how I yearn for diarrhea.

*Sore, dry, or ulcerated mouth* ... Yes, constant and painful.

*A pink-red colored urine. An irritated bladder.* Yes, peeing rosé into the hat is an around-the-clock activity, most certainly the result of the red devil.

*Flu-like symptoms including headaches, aching joints or muscles, a temperature, lethargy, and chills.* Yep.

*Fatigue.* Yes, this is the chemo big boy that no one escapes.

*In women, their periods may become irregular or stop. This will result in menopausal symptoms such as hot flashes, night sweats, and vaginal dryness.* Check. Check. And check.

I'd had a period in August but not as yet on September 15, Diagnosis Day. Perhaps my body didn't have the oomph to keep my cycle going with all those malignant cells reproducing like rabbits and killing off the last of the healthy eggs in my fifty-five-year-old ovaries. Not having to contend with a monthly period is a small plus while putting up with all of the other merciless Hyper-CVAD side effects.

This reading exhausts me but I have emails to answer, phone calls to return, and thank-you notes to write; but my fatigue and nausea mean a struggle to get pen to paper or fingers to laptop. I have no other option but to give myself the afternoon off and not die of guilt. Only my bladder remains active.

Dr. Greyz has thrown the book at me. Well, actually, it's the bag. And the further into treatment I fall, the further I am wrenched from all the activities that define me.

Seven days. Eight. More chemo, pints of blood, rescue meds.

Nine days. Ten. As chemo swaps place with my blood supply, I drift toward the sidelines of just being me. Immobilized in a hospital bed, I am a nauseated bystander in my own life. This role is not new—this is my second stint as bystander. The first happened when I was twelve and my father replaced me.

After he and my mother separated, my father married his secretary, Idel. It's so hackneyed to marry your secretary. He was her husband number three. Their marriage ceremony took place in Iowa; then they returned to California and tied the knot again when his divorce from my mother was final. Even at twelve, I thought that getting married twice to the same person in a couple of months sounded fishy. Much worse than his new wife—who was bordering on obese and had gums as long as her teeth—Idel had a six-year-old daughter, Stacy, from her second marriage, or maybe her first. I'm not sure. Within months, my father adopted Stacy—who was heavy like her mother and had a lazy left eye—and my replacement was complete. I'd been discarded. It took me decades to get over his abandonment. No. Maybe I never did.

## Chapter 20 - Fifty-Fifty Odds

DAY ELEVEN. DR. GREYZ STOPS by early this evening. Dan and I are watching the news. Well, Dan is watching the news; I am staring at the television. I hear voices but don't understand the words; even the pictures make no sense. My mind is a long way away in an encasing fog.

After greeting us, Dr. Greyz says, "Your vitals are strong. The Hyper-CVAD is destroying many cancer cells. Your progress, it is good."

I nod.

"There is something I must tell you," she says.

I am now alert. My body tenses, as if readying for another blow. Dr. Greyz takes a half-step toward me.

"After you have completed the chemo, you will need a bone marrow transplant."

I glance at Dan who frowns.

"In a situation as serious as yours, with nearly complete bone marrow involvement, it is almost certain that the cancer will come back and quickly."

I reach for Dan's hand.

"What will that entail?" he asks.

"The first thing is to find a donor. Do you have siblings?"

"Yes, two brothers."

"Oh, good. Any sisters?"

"No."

Dan looks at me sideways with a questioning expression.

"After you have finished the chemo, and are in remission, we will send them testing kits to determine if either of them is a match for you."

Dan reaches for the TV remote to turn off the set but hits the wrong button and the sound blares. The three of us flinch.

"Sorry," he says.

"What are the chances for a match?" I ask.

"Twenty-five percent for each sibling."

"That's it?"

"There may be a match in the international database of donors, but an unrelated donor can cause problems for you."

"So, with two brothers I have a fifty-fifty chance of a match?"

"Yes."

I'm on the verge of tears and blink my eyes.

"I am sorry to deliver this news, but I think you should know. I would rather tell you than you read it on the Internet." She pauses and puts her hand over mine. "Don't worry. Two brothers are good. I'll be back tomorrow."

"Thank you," I whisper as Dr. Greyz exits the room.

I look at Dan. His eyes are narrowed and he is clearly troubled.

"What was that about?" he asks.

"I didn't know about a bone marrow transplant either."

"I know. I'm sorry. But—"

"What do you mean?" I interrupt.

Dan sighs. "You didn't mention your third brother."

I toss the cotton blanket to the end of the bed.

"I haven't seen Johnny in thirty years. Haven't spoken to him in twenty-something. He's disappeared."

"You can't give up before you've started. You—we—might be able to find him."

"We've got Randy and Tom and the database."

"That's only fifty percent, and the database is risky."

"Johnny's gone. Believe me. He was into drugs for a long time. He might not even be alive."

Dan lets out a long breath. My hands are clenched; his insistence makes me anxious. I'm afraid to even think about finding Johnny and seeing the person he might be.

"I don't know if he survived backstreet deals or overdose. You didn't know him."

"No, I didn't, but wouldn't he try and save your life if he could?"

I shrug. "I don't know, I'm not sure what *I've* ever done for *him*."

"What do you mean?"

"When Johnny was thirteen, my mother phoned me and said, 'Johnny should live with you. You should raise him.' I was nineteen, a student at San Francisco City College and barely supported myself with a part-time cocktail waitressing job. It was all I could do to not get screwed over every day by life and strangers. I had a tiny studio apartment; there was nowhere for him to even sleep."

"It's ridiculous that Beverly asked you to be a mom to a teenager."

"She said he was a handful, distrustful, and emotionally distant."

"Sounds like a lot of kids at thirteen," says Dan.

"And maybe he was, but Beverly would never take responsibility for the harm she'd done to him. I always blamed her for making him into a wounded and reclusive kid. Her treatment of him could even be why he got into drugs—anything to escape reality."

"Honey, you couldn't have done anything."

"Maybe not, but I felt guilty and kept asking myself, *What did I ever actually do for Johnny? What would he say if I asked him?*"

"Stop blaming yourself."

"I wonder if he knows that I defended him a thousand times about how Beverly mistreated him? He was so young; he may have never been aware. And what did all that wrangling get us? I didn't try to visit Johnny after he'd been kicked out. I was already living in San Francisco. I called and wrote, a little, until he vanished, but I could have done more. I guess."

"And what would that have been? *Nothing* is what you could have done. You were a kid yourself and getting no help from anyone. You've got to give yourself a pass on this one. It was not your responsibility."

I gaze out the window but can't let the question go: W*hat did I do for Johnny*—even though life was roughing me up at the time and I was barely hanging on myself.

1970. I WAS NINETEEN. It was after 2 AM, and the bar where I worked as a cocktail waitress had closed. Another waitress needed a ride home and I offered to take her.

*"Hey, Susie can you swing back around and pick me up?" asked Clyde, the bartender, counting up the night's take, "My car's in the shop."*

*I was tired and wanted to go home, but he was my boss and I couldn't really say no. Twenty minutes later I got back to the club and knocked. Clyde opened the door and locked it behind me. The lights were dim and the bar smelled of stale smoke. A jazzy instrumental played on the sound system.*

*"I'm almost done."*

*I sighed, exasperated.*

*"You want a drink?" Clyde asked.*

*"No."*

*He grabbed my arms and pulled me to the floor. He tried to kiss me; I wrenched my head around. The thought of kissing him enraged and repulsed me. The smell of alcohol on his breath made my stomach turn. The carpet felt damp, almost mossy, on my bare arms.*

*"What's the matter?"*

*"Get off."*

*All of his weight was on top of me as he pulled up my skirt.*

*"Come on."*

*I shouted, "Go to hell!"*

*He was not a big man—only my height— and I found strength I didn't know I had. I was not going to be raped. I went for his throat and squeezed as hard as I could. He pried my hands away.*

*"Jesus, you must be a virgin," said Clyde.*

*"You bastard." I pushed him off and ran.*

I called the owner of the club the next day and was told that Clyde had done this before but he'd been there for ten years and was too valuable to lose. My resignation was accepted. After several days, the bruises and carpet burns on my arms and legs started to fade and I began to put the disgusting episode out of my mind. I was proud that I'd fought him off. I was more angry than anything else. The bigger problem was that the loss of this job began a long search for another one. After a number of fruitless interviews, I was getting frantic. Asking my parents for help was never an option, even though I was becoming financially desperate.

The Classified Ad: *Cocktail Waitress. Elite, private club. No experience necessary.*

*Topless* is what they were saying. But as a full-time college student, I couldn't find a part-time job that would pay enough to support myself. Seeing no other option, I called. The guy said he'd meet me at a phone booth on the corner of Lombard and Octavia streets. From there, we'd walk the couple of blocks back to my apartment in the Marina. I'd told my downstairs neighbor about this sordid job interview and asked her to come running if she heard me pound on the floor.

The day was overcast. He was there when I arrived on the busy corner. We shook hands. He looked innocent enough and maybe in his late twenties. Not much taller than I, he was clean shaven and wore a cheap-looking tan suit. I felt almost as sorry for him as I did for myself. Small talk was difficult. "How long have you been in this tawdry business?" wasn't the best of openers.

We climbed the stairs to my third-floor apartment, and I left the door unlocked behind us in case I needed help. He asked me to take off my shirt and bra, which I did in the bedroom. Topless, I walked into the living room, and he said I was hired. He handed me an address on a slip of paper. Show up that night at eight.

I didn't.

I eventually got a job at David's Delicatessen on Geary Street. It was brutal. David was a concentration camp survivor with a number tattooed on his forearm. He wore his shirt sleeves rolled up so the number was always visible. He despised everyone, especially those women employees who might have a few drops of German blood running through their veins. But I had to have money and stuck with it.

I hated thinking about the assault and the dismal little topless tryst and have put them far behind me. I've never told Dan. Guilty is how I felt about both of those shameful episodes. Like so many things, I blamed myself for getting into those jams. I blamed myself for doing nothing to help Johnny. I knew his home life was hellish, yet all I could do was fight with my mother about his treatment, which did nothing to make her love him.

IT'S GETTING DARK OUTSIDE. Across the courtyard, lights have come on in other patient rooms. Fifty-fifty odds. Not the best. Not the worst. But if Tom or Randy aren't a match, what will I do? I don't even know if Johnny's alive. He could be anywhere. Nowhere. And if I found him, which is probably impossible, would he speak to me, would he turn me down if I asked for his help? What if he's burned out? An addict? Homeless? I can't think about it anymore. Tom or Randy will be my match. They have to be.

# Chapter 21 - Johnny's Early Life, 1960–1986

"JOHNNY, GET IN HERE," yelled my mother.

Every morning it was the same. My sister and brothers had left for school. The air in the kitchen was thick with stale smoke.

"Sit down."

My mother glared at me as I sat across the Formica table from her. Cold in my cotton pajamas, I wrapped my arms around myself.

"Do you know why you're here?"

I nodded.

"Why? she barked.

"Because Dad made you do something."

"Yes. He forced me and you are what happened. A big mistake. Unwanted."

I looked down at my legs and tried not to cry. I always tried not to cry.

"And you will never amount to anything. Anything. Do you hear me?"

"Yes."

"Nothing more than a useless burden."

She lit another cigarette and for a moment was behind a thin cloud. I hated the sharp, sour smell of those cigarettes. She glanced at the kitchen clock. It was getting close to the time that she would go back into her bedroom to watch her soap opera. Then, I could leave the table. I pushed my chair back.

"You're not going anywhere."

She left the room and returned with an old woolen coat that my brothers had worn. She had large safety pins in her hand.

"Get up."

I stood.

She thrust it at me. "Put this on."

When the coat was around me, she pinned it closed with the safety pins and took me by the arm out the back door. She pulled me across the grass to the rusty, old swing set.

"Sit down and stay there."

She walked back into the house and slammed the door behind her.

I started to tremble and shake. I was freezing cold. Then, everything went black and I disappeared into a frozen, pitch-dark void. I don't know for how long.

Besides the constant punishments I received at my mother's hands, I was also a target for bullying by neighborhood kids and schoolmates. I wore thick glasses and looked like a nerd.

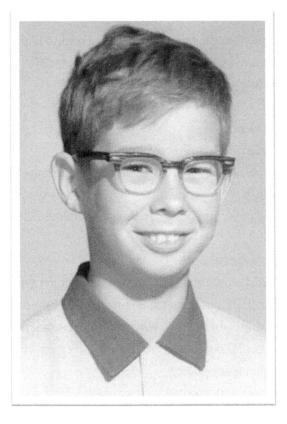

*Johnny, Age 8*

Because I wasn't accepted by my peers, I had to find somewhere else and lost myself in learning about the natural world. My face was always in a library book; I wanted to be a botanist, a herpetologist, or an entomologist. At nine years old, I was reading and comprehending college-level material in the biological subjects I loved. But at every step, I was dissuaded, and even ridiculed, by our mother and later Grandad Tom about my passion for nature. Even my teachers seemed to stand between me and my dreams. They had required subjects to teach that didn't include the study of the taxonomy, food sources, migration patterns, and life cycle of the Lepidoptera species (butterflies and moths) that fascinated me. But, by the fourth grade, I knew all of this—for every Lepidoptera in Southern California—plus, the birds and reptiles and small animals. I was an encyclopedia, as it turned out, of only minimally useful information.

# Chapter 22 - The Buddha, Pot, and a Visit from Randy

AS A SIXTEEN-YEAR-OLD POT-SMOKING, Buddhist-yogi surfer, I was *persona-non-grata* in my mother's and Grandad Tom's eyes. Grandad was one of those older people who became increasingly bitter with life and was never quite the same after his wife, Sophie, died eight years earlier. After her death, he moved in with us into our suburban Los Angeles home. Susie was already a student at U. C. Berkeley studying to become someone successful. I was exploring Eastern religion and the Southern California surf breaks. She and I lived in different worlds and rarely talked. I had little in common with Tom or Randy, either.

For a dollar, I bought a cheap, plaster Buddha from a friend's garage sale, mass produced in Tijuana of all places. I tinted the Buddha's face, feet, and hands with a pale bronze glaze to reflect the Buddha's possible Northern Nepalese heritage and repainted his faded purple robe into a pale orange, the color of renunciation in the Eastern Traditions. I placed the refreshed Buddha under the Chinese pear tree in our back yard.

One summer afternoon, I was lying under the tree in *Shavasana*—the dead man's pose. My long, wavy hair spread out on the grass around my head; I wore a white cotton tunic over gray sweatpants. My feet were bare. I heard someone approach and opened my eyes. Grandad leaned over me and frowned. "That plaster statue is nothing but a false idol. No one should worship it."

I startled and sat up. Grandad was ruddy, had pattern baldness, his eyes were perpetually squinted making him look angry, defensive, and ready to argue; he was twenty pounds overweight. I put my hands to my chest in the posture of *namaste*, knowing that there was no meeting place between us, no matter how hard I tried to be compassionate.

"Buddhists don't worship idols. We just use the image of the Buddha to be reminded to practice kindness in our daily lives."

"It's an ungodly idol." Grandad turned and walked away.

I lay back into *Shavasana*.

The Buddha had the strange habit of tipping over. I thought this impromptu lying on his side asana/yogic posture seemed, well, unnatural for the plaster statue. *Hadn't the Enlightened One transcended all of these yogic efforts shortly before his illumination under the Bodhi tree near Bodhgaya?*

Early one morning, I stood at the kitchen sink and looked out the window to see Grandad tip the statue over with his foot. I was sorely tempted to go outside and let him know I'd seen what he'd done, but I didn't. The Buddha would have simply smiled.

But Beverly and Grandad weren't done with me yet. They'd cooked up a scheme that was supposed to deter me from all things Buddhistic.

"We are going to send you to Thailand," warned Beverly.

"When?" I asked, thrilled by the prospect.

"I am talking about a one-way ticket and no way back. You will die over there! You don't even speak the language!" she said.

"I'm ready. Anytime."

I was sadly disappointed that nothing ever came of it. One day, shortly thereafter, the Buddha disappeared from under the pear tree.

There were many divisions between my mother and me: Eastern religion, my difficulties in school, and my collection of reptiles in the garage, which Beverly ultimately forced me to get rid of. But it was my use of drugs, cannabis mainly, that became our biggest issue. Funny though, she allowed Tom and Randy to smoke the stuff without raising a finger, or an eyebrow. Beverly said that their use of pot was okay because they kept their grades up, while I did not.

"I'll buy you beer, a six pack at a time, if you quit smoking pot," she said.

"I don't care about beer. Cannabis is way more interesting than alcohol."

She constantly went through my pockets, looked under my bed, in dusty boxes of old board games on closet shelves, obtuse nooks and crannies in the garage, anywhere she could wage her special vendetta to eradicate the pot. On occasion, she would succeed and find my prized stash, which for some peculiar reason she ferreted away in her underwear drawer (which I found and happily stole back).

Waving around a discovered baggie of pot, she said, "I am going to call the police on you."

"That's exactly what should happen," agreed Grandad. "Maybe moldering around in a jail cell for a good long while will teach you a lesson."

I feigned disinterest but was disturbed. I wouldn't put it past them calling the cops and still had undiscovered stashes in several places around the house.

"I'm not the only one taking drugs around here." I turned toward my mother. "What about the decades you've been swallowing opiates, tranquilizers, and antidepressants? You don't think that's drug abuse?"

"I am prescribed those drugs legally and for medical reasons, while what you are doing is illegal! And that makes you a criminal."

"People who drink at the end of the day aren't one bit superior to the person who smokes weed."

"Weed," Grandad sneered.

"People who have a drink are not breaking the law. That's a very big difference," said my mother.

The room was too warm—stifling, like my life.

"And you need a haircut. How will you ever get a job looking like that?"

I pushed my heavy, shoulder-length hair behind my ears. I'd be graduating high school in two days. I hadn't considered what I was going to do but had applied for a job as a groundskeeper at a local nursing home. I didn't know if I wanted the job or not.

"Is your high school even going to let you graduate looking like that?" asked Beverly.

"Don't worry. You don't have to come."

"I wasn't planning on it."

I shrugged in relief and disappointment.

"If you got a haircut, maybe," said Beverly.

"Don't count on it."

"Don't talk to your mother that way," yelled Grandad.

"Or what?"

"*Or what*, is that you can walk right out that door and not come back."

I smiled and sensed freedom like a shark sensed blood. I was excited at how close it felt. This was just the push I needed. I glanced outside at the showy pear tree, my peaceful meditation spot. I would miss that. Little else.

The day before graduation, to which Beverly and Grandad did not come, I moved in with Walter, a high school surfer buddy. Walt's mom had gone off to live in San Clemente with her new boyfriend, and Walter had "inherited" the house. I was there for about a year, two 18-year-old surfer types smoking pot, growing "magic mushrooms," *Psilocybin Cubensis,* in a bedroom closet, and taking LSD and peyote. No adult supervision and complete freedom. Well, not complete freedom as I did get the job at the nursing home. But overall, this situation suited me just fine. I loved to hike on full moon nights in the Whittier Hills while under the influence of Shroom Booms, or peyote.

Walter and I were starting one of those hikes when the police spotted us, caught me in possession of a couple grams of hashish, and carted me off to L.A. County Jail. Fourteen of the worst days of my life. As bad as it was, jail time didn't change the choices I continued to make—taking drugs and dealing them.

Two years later, in June of 1977, I was barely getting by and living in a run-down twelve-unit apartment complex a couple of blocks from the ocean.

Late one Friday afternoon, a party was getting underway on the top-floor patio of my building. The spring breeze was warm. North, to the Huntington Beach Pier, the ocean was glassy. I was happy there. I was liked and accepted; it felt good to me. While gazing at the rolling surf, I noticed someone appear on the rooftop. It was Randy. I hadn't seen him in two years. He didn't smile but walked directly toward me. We didn't touch. No hugs. No handshakes.

"I'm surprised to see you. How did you find me?" I asked.

"I met up with your surfer buddy, Walter. I asked him. He told me where you lived."

People were drinking beer and pot was being smoked. Randy accepted a beer but refused the joint. I accepted a beer as well. Randy frowned at me and refused to sit.

"You still surfing?" I asked.

"Yeah, but I didn't come here to talk about surfing."

"Everybody okay?"

"What do you care? You've tried to disappear."

I had no answer and looked down at my bare feet.

Randy sounded impatient, "What are you going to *do* with your life?"

I leaned backward on my heels. I felt defensive and thought, *why do I have to answer this?* Still, I hoped my brother might understand. I looked at him.

"Man, I worked a couple years in a convalescent hospital. I made friends with the patients, then watched them die. I'm done with that. I just wanna surf and take it easy."

"So, that's it, surf and take it easy? How are you going to support yourself?"

"I do odd jobs for the Hindu owners of a nearby motel, and I sell enough home-grown magic mushrooms to get by."

"Dealing drugs? That's a great future!"

I cringed and felt the old judgment again.

"I also write, draw, paint, and hang out with my buddies on the beach."

"But what are you going to *do?*"

"I'm doing it."

Randy shook his head, looked around at the other residents—all under thirty, long-haired, and disheveled—and said, "What a bunch of losers!"

I figured he included me in that group.

Randy took a long swig of beer, turned, and left. I felt relieved but defeated, rejected. I'd hoped, for one short moment, that my brother and I could be friends, but I knew that I'd never measure up to his expectations or be able to fall into society's march step of school, job, marriage, mortgage, and kids that Randy had signed up for. I simply wasn't that guy and I would pay for my outlier choices for the rest of my life.

WHILE I WAS LIVING MY surfing and magic mushroom days, I became friends with two girls in my apartment building who decided to make a pet project of reconnecting me with Susie, with whom I hadn't spoken in years. I didn't know how many.

I called them The Doughnut Girls because of their daily habit of gorging on a box of doughnuts and then bemoaning the binge to anyone within hearing distance. The Doughnut Girls went to great lengths to put me and my sister back in touch. I never knew how they pulled it off. I didn't have a telephone at the time and had to use the apartment manager's.

During this—our last—conversation, it was likely 1984, I told my sister that I worked as the maintenance person at a building in Huntington Beach and received an apartment and enough money to buy groceries. I also grew and sold psilocybin mushrooms to increase my income.

While I was honest about my dealing, I'm sure she didn't like it. She suggested I find something lawful, like working at a pet store, which made me feel judged. I'd had enough condemnation from the rest of the family. Thank you.

I said that I also spent a fair amount of time surfing and exploring the nearby beaches, including Swami's Point, where the ashram for the followers of Bhagwan Shree Rajneesh was located high on the bluffs overlooking the ocean. During the past year, I'd become a devoted *sannyasin* in the movement, believing that the Bhagwan was Enlightened.

I told her that I might give away my meager possessions and move to the mother-ship ashram in Oregon, joining the sect of the Bhagwan.

"Isn't that the guy who is chauffeured around in Rolls Royces and has a collection of diamond-studded Rolex watches?" Susie asked.

"Yeah."

"Does that bother you?"

"No. He is Enlightened and deserves everything that comes into his life."

My sister sighed. With this last conversation, our already frayed relationship further unraveled.

Simply put, we had no common ground. Sometimes, love is not enough.

I gave her the phone number of the apartment manager and my address. We wrote a couple times until a year later when I moved again and didn't let her know where I'd gone. I honestly didn't know what good it would do. I was out of touch with the whole family and it seemed for the best.

Until two years later when that changed.

# Chapter 23 - The Private Eye

"JOHNNY?"

"Yeah?"

"It's John, your father."

I scowled and wondered, *Was this some sick, practical joke?*

"Who?"

"Your father." There was a trace of impatience, or was it embarrassment, in the man's voice on the phone.

I heard a tone, an inflection I recognized, and wished this was a deranged prank.

"I'm surprised," I said.

"I understand. I'm in L.A. We should meet."

"How did you find me?"

I looked out my second-floor window onto the parched and dusty garden of philodendron, bird of paradise, and jacaranda trees. The flowers of the jacaranda had dropped and become purple stains where tenants had walked over them for days. It was fall and hadn't rained since March.

"I hired a private investigator."

"Why?"

"Because I'm your father. Dammit."

I wanted to ask, *since when*, but didn't.

"How about tomorrow?" John asked.

"Sure. I guess you know my address."

In the kitchen, I opened a beer. I was unhinged by this out-of-left-field phone call, but also relieved as I'd heard from one of my psilocybin customers that a detective had been asking around about me. Now I knew that the detective wasn't working for the Narco Division of the Huntington Beach Police Department but for dear old Dad who was probably just trying to clear his own conscience by seeing his youngest son who he hadn't bothered with for more than two decades. Thinking about this visit put me into a foul and apprehensive mood. I slugged back the beer, then opened another.

About noon the next day, the doorbell rang and there he stood. I felt as if I was looking at a stranger, which, essentially, he was. His jaw was tight as he tried to smile. Neither of us succeeded at this. The sight of my father made me feel wary, even afraid.

We shook hands and I realized I had no recollection of my father ever touching me.

"Come in."

John walked past me and I waited for the rank smell of cigarettes and alcohol, but there was only a trace of cologne. He was older, of course, but looked much the same. His hair was still dark but he wore it in a crew cut now—the thick waves that I'd inherited from him, gone—his goatee and temples were mostly gray. His posture was straight, his body still slender. As he moved into the room, I felt the same ripple of terror that I had as a child when he came home bellowing drunk, which was the only way I remembered him.

Christine sat on our thrift shop couch. I introduced her as my girlfriend, and, without standing, she said, "I'm glad to meet Johnny's father."

Of course, she'd asked me about him, but I'd had little to say other than the basic details of alcoholism, abandonment, and divorce. Having issues with her own estranged Roman Catholic father, she didn't press it. I never expected my father to show up, and discussion of him had only happened a couple of times.

John shook Christine's hand, smiled, and said, "Nice to meet you."

She then made a quick exit saying she was off to work.

John looked around, then out the window, a crease between his eyebrows.

"I've seen better maintained apartment complexes."

I was both insulted and at the same time proud of my alternative lifestyle.

"Yeah, well, it's called The Animal House. It's where the poorer young people end up. Everything here in Huntington Beach is getting gentrified and is way too expensive. We don't have a choice. We might not even be able to stay here much longer."

Why had my father had gone to all the trouble and expense to track me down? I knew he wouldn't approve of me: the long hair, old jeans, a tie-dye tee shirt, and the crummy apartment. It was obvious my father didn't like what he saw.

Anxious to keep things moving, I said, "Let's get out of here."

I directed him to a nearby lunch spot where the beach crowd hung out. Picnic tables and benches needed a paint job; salt and pepper shakers needed a good scrub—not the kind of place that he would have frequented. The cafe had a satisfying, greasy smell. We found seats in the back.

John asked, "So what do you do, Johnny? Or do you go by John now?"

"Johnny's fine. I'm the maintenance supervisor at a retirement community for wealthy ambulatory folks who basically take care of themselves."

John looked out the window, blinked, and shook his head ever so slightly. I felt judged and worried that the whole lunch would go like this—one tacit criticism after the next. I wanted to bolt.

"Well, I'm real happy you've found such a pretty gal."

His comment about Christine felt sincere.

"She's a good person."

"So, I guess you never went to college?"

"No."

"Your sister and brothers went. Why didn't you?"

"It wasn't for me."

"I wish I could have helped you, with tuition or whatever."

I was confused. If he'd wanted to help, why didn't he? Had he helped my sister or brothers? As vague and flimsy as the statement was, I was warmed by the affection contained in it. If he really wanted to help me, it was a first.

"My job suits me. The residents are kind and appreciate what I do for them. I don't need anything else."

"You have your future to think about."

"Christine and I are fine."

I waited for another objection, but he seemed to be done with the subject.

"I hope you don't mind if I talk with you, man to man," said John.

"I don't mind." But I did.

John looked down at his hands and then back at me. "It's not completely unfair to say that all of the problems in our family were Beverly's fault."

I shifted in my seat and my neck grew hot. I had no desire to hear any of this and even though Beverly mistreated me for years, I doubted that *all* of the problems were her fault. I remembered again my father's immense and explosive anger.

"I wanted a son to name John. Your mother didn't want any more children. Perhaps I shouldn't have done what I did, but … you're here now."

I tightened and recalled the abuse I got from her in the mornings at the kitchen table when she told me I was only here because my father forced her.

"I should have taken you. But your mother wouldn't let me."

"That's funny. She told me that she'd asked you many times and you refused."

"That's not true. I would have."

"Hardly matters, does it?"

I felt again the echoing sadness of my childhood that I'd tried so hard to forget. Hallucinogenics, meditation, getting lost in the wonders of the natural world, and surfing had helped me put those memories away. Now, with my father sitting across from me, I was face to face with them again.

John sighed. "Maybe not. Long time ago."

I was relieved when our food arrived.

"Do you know that I quit drinking twenty years ago?"

"No. How was I supposed to know that? Do you want a trophy?"

John straightened in his chair. His eyes widened. "I deserved that. I was a sick S.O.B."

"I'm sorry. I guess you had an illness." My anger with my father abated as quickly as it had flared.

"It was complicated. But that's not an excuse," he said.

We ate in silence.

Then John asked, "Do you drink?"

"The occasional beer."

"Is that it?"

"Pretty much."

I had no intention of telling him about my nightly joint and wine, or my and Christine's regular sampling of mushrooms and peyote.

"Take it from me, booze isn't worth it."

"I don't rely on it."

"Don't. You'll be sorry."

"Do you see Susie? Talk to her?" I asked.

"Yeah. We're both up north. I see her every couple months. She's fine. Married. Has a daughter. She works too hard."

I wasn't sure if that meant I didn't.

"I really don't communicate with Tom. Neither of us ever tried to connect, but Randy's great. Married. Two kids. He's a high school history teacher. History, that's something he and I share. Do you like history?"

"I'm more into biology. I also study Buddhist psychology and religion."

Once more, John looked out the window. He didn't say so, but I figured the words going through his head were, *Great. Just great. That's the way to get ahead!*

"Okay, then, another topic. I own a company," he said.

"Oh?"

"An engineering operation. I could give you a job."

"I'll think about it."

A job at my father's firm might be the last thing I would want, still I felt a warmth from him that I'd never known. He'd just offered me something and it seemed like a very big, and maybe even sincere, gesture.

The music got turned up and the café was getting noisy. John leaned in closer to me. "How long since you've seen your sister or brothers?"

"A few years. I don't know." I wasn't going to elaborate on Randy's last finger-shaking visit.

John looked wistful. "I'm proud of Randy. He's so good-looking, quite an athlete too."

I saw the pride in my father's eyes and stung with a flash of jealousy.

"I think we should go right now and drive down to see him," said John, his voice quickening.

"No thanks." Once again, I felt the way I had the last time I saw Randy: always lacking, coming up short on any measurement my family had for me.

"It's only an hour. I'd like you to see how well he's doing."

"I have to work."

When we pulled up in front of my apartment, John reached into the breast pocket of his sports coat. "Here, I want you to have this."

I looked at the two-hundred-dollar bond. "You don't need to."

"I want to. Take it."

"Thank you."

He wrote his home address and phone number on the back of his business card and said, "Call me if you need anything."

We shook hands. I wasn't clear on why my father had looked me up. The meeting left me feeling sad for all that had never been between us, yet subtly yearning to see him again. Maybe next time would be easier. He would like Christine. She would make it smoother between us.

At Christmas that year, Christine and I visited San Francisco. I phoned my father, who lived nearby, to say hello. I was hoping for an invitation to his home. It didn't come. Our conversation was short, but we promised to stay in touch. While I wouldn't know it for many years, my father died the next July. That Christmas call was the last time we spoke.

# Chapter 24 - Susan 2005

AFTER TWELVE DAYS OF "house arrest" and completion of the first round of Course A Hyper-CVAD, I am sprung from the chemo ward. It is heaven to have the IV pulled out of my hand and the Huber needle out of my chest. To simply move without bondage makes me giddy. When the orderly pushes my wheelchair out of the hospital and I hear the heavy glass doors whoosh behind us, I raise my chin and say, "Yes!" Compared with the dry, lackadaisical atmosphere of the hospital, the cold outside air buzzes like blue neon. After two deep breaths, I feel as if I've thrown back a double Sapphire martini.

Today is the first of nine days at home before the start of Course B—nine days of living a normal life—when I can think about throw pillows and area rugs, what to wear instead of a hospital gown, and how many billable hours I might rack up during these days of freedom. My clients have emailed notes of caring and concern that moved me with their compassion, and I want to get back to work.

Some people might be composing bucket lists, calling everyone from high school, or pricing burial plots. Others of us are expert at the game of denial and hang onto old, controlling habits with every muscle fiber even when life, or fate, has walloped us out of all semblance of the norm.

Like a salmon, I swim furiously back upstream toward my previous life, toward what I know as home, toward the woman I know as myself.

This morning, I wield a blow dryer over my clean, wet hair. Half of it flies in all directions around the bathroom, the rest clings to my head in exhausted little patches.

Elspeth walks in, and I turn off the dryer.

"Geez, Mom."

"I look like one of those poor, mangy dogs in Mexico."

"Oh. I'm sorry." Elspeth runs her hand down her long blond ponytail.

I sigh.

"So, what's going on?" she asks.

"Sometimes I don't know if I'm worth all of this."

"This what?"

"Effort. Upheaval. The emotional drain on everyone." I wave the quiet blow dryer around.

"You're talking crazy," says Elspeth.

"I guess it's stupid."

"It's not stupid, but it's not the right question."

"What's the right question?"

"You need to ask me if I will fix that weird hair-do thing you have going on."

"Yeah, I'm sorry." I laugh. "That's what I mean."

We hug for a long minute before Elspeth kisses my cheek and goes downstairs. From the dining room, she wrangles a chair outside and tries to level it onto our still dirt-clod backyard. I carry a towel and scissors and sit in the sunlight on this brisk and cloudless October morning. The rosemary—in a pot outside the back door—smells pungent, like a Creosote Bush.

We have no mirror. The sharp blades close with a metallic snip. Like my recent life, strands of hair drift and tumble across the churned-up yard then disappear.

"I haven't told anyone about this, but sometimes things look different," I say.

"What do you mean?" asks Elspeth.

"Colors. Green is so green. The sky kind of quivers. Everything is intense and alive."

"Sounds cool. A little hallucinogenic."

"I don't see it all the time."

"Is it good, or not?"

"Very good."

Hair floats across the yard.

"It makes me feel connected. Like I'm in the sky, the trees, the hills. There's no separation between me and the whole world. It's blissful. I don't know. It feels like I'm everything. I sound so dumb."

"You don't sound dumb. I think it's your vision. For healing. Hold onto it."

"Yes. I need that." My voice breaks as I struggle for a breath against the pressure on my chest.

"Dad and I will always be here. So will a lot...." Elspeth begins to cry.

I could double over in pain when I see my daughter cry. I stand and hold her, both of us now in tears.

Dan, who has just come home from getting his own hair cut, calls out from the doorway, "I told my barber you might be losing your hair and she loaned me a Norelco."

I look over at his smiling face and ask, "A what?"

"An electric clipper."

Dan always comes to the rescue.

"What's going on?" he asks.

"Elspeth and I are having a crying fest."

He bounds over the lumpy earth and the three of us have a laughing, sobbing, family hug.

"Thank you," I say.

"It's just a loaner."

"I wasn't talking about the Norelco."

Back inside, Elspeth eases the no-nonsense clipper over my head and gives me a loving buzz cut. I touch what's left of my hair. "It's soft and feels like puppy fur."

I smile. Dan takes photos and Elspeth says how good I look without hair. And I feel pretty—not me, but pretty.

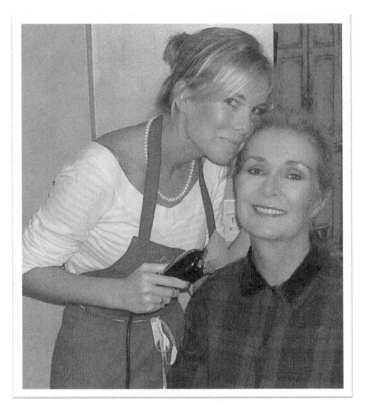

*Elspeth and Susan*

We go shopping and I buy a sexy wig, more J. Lo than Andie McDowell, as well as a blonde Martha Stewart version. In the fun-house-like atmosphere of the wig and costume shop, full of Halloween paraphernalia, I step into another persona and leave myself further behind. But I'm not all gone. Not yet. I promise—for Dan and for Elspeth—that I won't just give up. No. I won't.

Hyper-CVAD makes food taste like over-ripe wood—ropy and fibrous—but wood, from Mars with a bitter, metallic after bite. Rotting Martian wood isn't easy to describe but it's a cinch to decline. Even at home, on this break from chemo, most food is still appalling.

Its bizarre and off-putting taste and texture leads to a cancer bonus: weight loss without trying. For those of us who tend toward the pudge, effortless (well, not exactly) weight loss is a real bonus.

After a couple of days, all of my abdominal and lower body squishiness from Round A has vanished. My face is no longer puffy. This morning in the mirror, my naked body is hairless—some women pay a lot for this effect— and I say to Dan, "I look as though I've just spent way too long at a spa that specializes in waxing."

He groans.

Yes, Hyper-CVAD is a go-for-broke bitch. But even with the physical and emotional bruising that life is currently throwing at me, I will be alright. Even if food tastes like metallic wood. Even if I'm bald. Even if my future will be in a chemo ward, I'll be okay. I'm tough—like an ocean buoy in tumultuous water—I take what comes and remain upright, even if I bob and lean now and again.

# Chapter 25 - Full Code

CHECKING INTO THE ADMISSIONS DEPARTMENT today for the beginning of Course B Hyper-CVAD, I must fill out an Advance Directive—the "What-Ifs" paperwork—asking which measures I want taken to keep me from dying.

I chew at my nails and wonder why today and not earlier. Am I now in more danger than during my first admission when I was on the brink of a heart attack or a brain aneurism?

The light in the cramped office is white and too bright. It's hot and airless. The wooden table may be the hardest thing I've ever rested my wrists on. Laurie and I sit with papers strewn in front of us. The clerk, likely bored from having been through this drill a thousand times before, eyes me from over her glasses.

"Ask if there's something you don't understand."

*What if I don't understand anything?*

Let's see … a feeding tube versus antibiotics. Antibiotics. Of course. A feeding tube? I don't even know exactly what a feeding tube is. Sure, I've heard of it, but how much surgery is involved, is it painful, and does it come out? How can I even answer this feeding tube question? *Temporary* life support or the *likelihood* of not recovering. Temporary sure. How long is temporary? *Eventualities* of not being able to talk or enjoy life. Do eventualities come with a percentage?

I look at Laurie, "Eventualities or likelihoods? Red or white? Rare or medium?"

*Sorry*, she mouths.

Tissue and organ donation choices. Health care agents. Yes. No. Unsure. Leave it up to my doctors and loved ones. *What if they disagree?* My mind reels at language and subtle choices that I am certain will not apply to me. I have never had to instruct anyone to pull the plug. Other than putting down a sick dog, I've never had to make any other heartbreaking decisions: to divorce or stay together, to cheat or remain faithful. I'm certain that I will be spared the wrenching scenarios described in the Advance Directive as well.

No. I am not going to die. Still, I check the FULL CODE box on the paperwork. Hell yes. I want Code Blue broadcast all over the hospital's loudspeakers. I want the crash cart with the paddles and a half dozen docs rushing into my room—if anything goes wrong. But it won't. I sign and date in black ink.

With paperwork finalized, Laurie helps me settle into 522, my same private room. She stays while Mike, a nurse on the floor, accesses my VAP. More accurately, tries to access my VAP. He does the necessary cleansing of the area then asks, "Ready?"

"Sure."

"Here we go." He pushes the Huber into my chest and then says, "Hmm."

"Hmm" is an ominous sound coming from the person sticking needles into your body. I glance down and see that he's not gotten any blood return, indicating that he has not entered the vein. He stares at the device then smiles.

"A little temperamental today, aren't we?" he asks, addressing the Huber.

I look at his fingers, which are fat. Aren't people with fat fingers less dexterous? He begins to re-adjust the Huber. Re-adjust is a kind and delicate term to describe the process of pulling the needle most of the way out, re-inserting at another angle, and applying more pressure. Oh dear. Still no blood return.

"All of these are a little different," he says.

*What? That's crazy. How can one Huber needle be any different than another?*

I'm squirmy. Laurie rolls her eyes and shakes her head. Being stuck in the chest makes me feel so vulnerable—like an insect specimen being pinned to a slab of Styrofoam. The arm is an extremity; the chest is our core. A nice guy and talkative, I am tempted to ask Mike to stop chattering and pay attention to the task at hand: perforating my chest. But I don't. This is a small detail and I won't make a fuss. I've been very careful to keep all of the nurses squarely on my side and I silently put up with the piercing. After three needle sticks, he finally gets blood out of the Huber and saline into the VAP. I am not unhappy to see him go. Laurie and I chat for a while until I convince her to get on with her day.

Shortly after she leaves, Mike returns, as upbeat as before.

"I've come to insert your IV."

A nearly audible groan escapes my lips.

"Could you please avoid the insides of my elbows since an IV there makes bending my arm and doing anything just about impossible?"

"Roger that."

He ties a tourniquet on my lower left arm and pushes on a vein. "Looks like a winner." He sticks and misses. He pulls the needle part way out and tries another angle. No luck. "Hmm," comes his second medical analysis of the situation.

Then another tourniquet, more Morse Code-like pumping to find a vein, and another stick. Misses again. "You sure have some wallflower veins in there," he jokes, "they just don't want to join the party."

He remains cheerful and unbowed.

"Let's try that right side," Mike says, undeterred by his abysmal lack of success.

He walks to the other side of the bed. Again, he attempts to oblige my request for an IV not inside the elbow area but after several tied tourniquets and lots of ineffectual thumping, he determines that I have no useable vein. He then ties the tourniquet above my right elbow, palpates the bend in my arm, and says, "Here she is. Third time's a charm." He sticks me and gets the vein but the placement of the IV—exactly where I don't want it—is such that I can't bend or use my right arm at all.

He smiles, gives me a thumbs up, and says in a confident tone, "You're all set now. Good to go, as they say."

*And just where is that supposed to be?*

He swaggers out of the room as if he'd just accomplished something of a personal best, which he very well might have.

Mike has just made me into a one-handed leftie. I pick up a pen and my notebook from the bedside table and try to write. Repeated efforts prove my left-handedness impossible. Not only is the task laborious; but after just a few lines, even I can't decipher what I've written. I had hoped to write thank-you notes to friends and neighbors who have brought us so many dinners but won't be able to until I have the use of my right hand.

As unexpected as it sounds, these days sequestered in the hospital can be busy: trying to journal (well, not post-Mike); receiving visitors; doing a minimal amount of client work; and cleaning up. I try very hard not to ask for help. I learned from my Course A hospitalization that preparing for the day was an effort, but a task I could accomplish. Showering was impossible because of all the apparatus attached to me. And with an IV (usually in my hand) bathing at the sink had to be done with only one hand—possible but not quick, and lots of ineffectual rinsing was required.

A further exasperation: the chemo pump squawks every time I move my right arm. Perhaps placement of the IV is creating a kink in the line. Breathing deeply, I tell myself that this hospital stint will only be four or five days. I'll find a way to accept the racket. Then the door opens and a woman enters introducing herself as the head charge nurse. The *jefa* R.N. says that placement of the IV and movement of my right arm are causing an interruption in the chemo drip. She taps around on my left hand and decides she will have no problem inserting another IV, which she does quickly and nearly painlessly. Now, I am free to use my right hand again, and the nurse and I smile at each other.

"Thanks," I say. She high-fives me and replies, "Anytime." Funny what can bring joy.

I write the notes. I email my clients thanking them for their concern and assure them I will keep critical aspects of their projects moving forward. Early in the afternoon I become fatigued and put my laptop down. I gaze out the window at the hospital roof, the gray vents and pipes that stand upright like a scattered battalion guarding the patients inside against an infantry of invading microbes led by the brilliant strategist, General Malignancy. (I have definitely been in this hospital too long.)

That evening, like all evenings, Dan comes to visit.

"I had to fill out an Advance Directive today."

His forehead creases. He looks worried.

"It was more subtle than I'd thought, with a lot of shalls and eventualities."

"I wish I'd been here."

"Me too. It wasn't easy." I sound crabby.

"I've got a job."

"I know that."

"Do you want me to go over it with you?"

"No. It's just paperwork. I asked for every damn thing to be done to save my life."

"That's right."

"I know I won't need any heroics but answering all those questions made me think about how much time I have left."

"Jesus."

Dan gazes out the window, his jaw is set.

"I'm not telling you to call the undertaker."

He looks back at me.

"Three things can happen. I am miraculously cured and die an old lady, or I get everything that Western medicine has to throw at me and am cancer-free for a few years. That's if I can find a bone marrow donor. Or the damn lymphoma comes right back."

"Honey, it won't come back."

I can feel my face settling into a *How do you know that?* expression.

"We both know that it can and does."

Dan reaches for my hand.

"We gotta be strong. Do what Dr. Greyz says. Stay the course."

*Easy for him*, I think.

"It'll be okay," he says.

"Glad you think so."

"What do you want me to say?"

"Nothing," I reply.

"Come on, Honey. Think about Elspeth. Think about me."

"You're right. I'm sorry."

"You're upset. I don't blame you."

*Why am I lashing out at my husband? He's so loyal and loving.* I calm down.

"I spoke with a woman a few days ago in the oncology waiting room. She's got MCL too and will get a transplant from her sister. She's also going through a divorce," I say.

"Wow, that's bad timing."

"When she told her husband about the cancer, he said to her, 'I didn't feel anything. That's when I knew I had to leave you.' Then he moved in with a woman twenty years younger than himself."

"God, that's heartless."

"I'm so lucky to have you," I say.

"I'm so lucky to have you."

"That seems like an overstatement at the moment, but I'll take it."

Dan climbs into bed and holds me until I fall asleep.

# Chapter 26 - My Dream House—Antithesis to the Advanced Directive

AFTER MORE THAN TWENTY-FIVE YEARS, Dan and I are still in love and deeply dependent on each other. I plan our social life and vacations. He opens jars. He fills my car with gas and takes it to the mechanic. I decorate.

Dan has never resisted my management of our finances and, luckily, money has been a fairly smooth ride. When we met, he had a $2,000 savings account and I still owed $2,000 on a student loan. Nice fit. Right?

We've spent the last quarter of a century working and saving to get to a place where we are approaching comfort. Not wealth, by any stretch, but we can take appliance repairs in stride and enjoy an annual, two-week vacation. We are also footing (most of) the bill for Elspeth to attend USC, a pricey, private university.

But there is one way I want to spend big that Dan does not: buying our (my) dream house. We've been in the same house for fifteen years. When we bought it, the neighborhood was a great place to raise our daughter. I figured we'd live there until Elspeth could drive, but I never planned to stay for the duration.

When we moved in, the house needed a ton of work, and Dan will gently remind me that we've upgraded virtually every square inch of it; he is not looking forward to doing that again. I get it.

I've dragged my good-natured husband to countless open houses. We've been in escrow a few times, but for one reason or another, the deal never went through.

When I start yammering about my fantasy house, Dan gets all philosophical and spiritual on me and recites *"The Chambered Nautilus"* by Oliver Wendell Holmes:

*"...Build thee more stately mansions, O my soul,*
*As the swift seasons roll!*
*Leave thy low-vaulted past!*
*Let each new temple, nobler than the last,*
*Shut thee from heaven with a dome more vast,*
*Till thou at length art free,*
*Leaving thine outgrown shell by life's unresting sea!"*

Dead, in other words.

The "shut thee from heaven with a dome more vast," line is the kicker. Dan can be so superior: indulgent of my house-hunting obsession, but superior. His is a more internal life, which he inherited from his dad. Years ago, when I asked my father-in-law if he had any goals, he said, "None that you can see." That struck me. Dan shares many of these sensibilities; and is currently reading Krishnamurti, for heaven's sake. Do people who read Krishnamurti yearn for stainless steel appliances, recycled glass countertops, and an open floor plan? I appreciate the irony of this in that at nineteen, I was also enthralled with Krishnamurti and read all of his books.

When Dan comes into room 522 this Sunday morning, I am pouring over the Real Estate Section of Houses for Sale. I love the smell of the ink and the feel of the crisp paper that promises, or at least makes possible, adventure, change. He sees the newspaper and rolls his eyes.

"I'm just looking."

"Kind of strange timing," he says.

"Why?"

"Maybe you need to put your energy into getting better."

"This," I rustle the newspaper, "makes me feel better."

Dan believes that my compulsion for change is a psychological flaw. Contentment is a goal instilled in him by his parents.

"Why can't you just be happy?" he asks.

"I am happy. Well, maybe not in this hospital room. But just because I dream of a new house, doesn't mean that I'm miserable."

Even I get tired of my own whining.

"All this churning," he says shaking his head.

(Imagine Gandhi trying to make a go of it with Leona Helmsley.)

"My dream house is life moving forward and has nothing to do with feeding tubes or not being able to walk or speak."

"Of course, I want you to have a place where you're happy."

"Here we go again with the happiness refrain."

"Well, isn't that it?"

"No. A new home is about being alive. Creating beauty. Writing chapters to life after cancer."

He gives me that face again that says, *I wish you could just be satisfied.*

I wonder if lymphoma will give me a perspective on the importance of this dream house. Maybe, maybe not. But I know myself. If I'm well, even halfway well, I won't give it up.

"Look whatever happens, you cannot use the money from my life insurance policy to buy your second wife her—or my—dream house. Absolutely, positively, not."

He smiles in spite of himself.

"Give us a kiss," I say, opening my arms.

# Chapter 27 - The Espresso Cart

IN CHINA, THE COLOR OF DEATH is white. Lifeless. Bloodless. Fierce. White is the color of my nightmare. Trapped in a building of bleached walls with sharp angles and identical corridors that have no end, my legs are heavy as marble as I try to outrun something huge and fixed on destroying me.

Waking, my fists are clenched and my heart pounds. The early morning sky is pallid, like the nightmarish hallways. Fearing that the dream will suck me back into those corridors, I struggle to sit up. After a soft knock, a nurse enters.

I wipe my wet face on the hot, rumpled sheets.

"I understand," says the nurse.

*How can she?*

She hands me four tablets. "These will make you feel better."

"What are they?"

"Dexamethasone."

"Dexa?"

"Methasone. A steroid. It'll lift your mood."

The D in Hyper-CVAD.

I know it isn't his fault, but I can't stop myself from griping at the man who brings in the sorry breakfast tray. "This coffee is terrible."

"You can get a latte in the cafeteria."

"A latte?"

"Yes, ma'am. There's an espresso cart on the first floor."

"Really? An espresso cart?" Delighted, I beam at him. "Thank you."

Pulling my pink wool cap over my bald head and putting on my bathrobe, I shove sunglasses onto my face, grab ten dollars, unplug the monitor, and maneuver the tree out the room and toward the elevator. I hope to ride solo, but no such luck. The people entering on the floors below glance at me, then find their shoes of particular interest. On the ground floor, the elevator door slides open to the smell of bacon, fried potatoes, and coffee. Real coffee. Chairs with metal feet scrape across the linoleum floor. The laughter and chatter make me move faster in my hospital socks with the little grippers on the bottom. At the sight of the coffee cart, I have to stop myself from shoving a raised fist into the air and shouting, "Yes." Giddy, I order a double latte with non-fat milk. The hissing of the espresso machine makes me shift my weight from side to side. The tip I leave is larger than the cost of the coffee. Returning upstairs takes more skill as I now have to move the hot latte from hand to hand. Back in my room, I hold onto my tiny luxury in a paper cup, take a sip and let the milky bitterness linger on my tongue. I whisper, "Thank you. Thank you."

The chemical combo of caffeine and dexamethasone dissolves my earlier, terrified frame of mind. I make up my face, send chirpy emails, and don't mind peeing in a hat one little bit. Drugs. Wow.

Lunch arrives: a dried-out turkey sandwich with two packets of bright yellow Heinz mustard, no lettuce, tomato, or pickle—my blood counts are too low. I can't eat raw fruits or vegetables that could be carrying microbes. Who cares? I'm starved and finish the sandwich, sloppy with both packets of mustard.

A couple hours later, depression and anxiety—like two old, weirdo boyfriends that I never want to see again—begin to creep around. My body becomes leaden and I struggle to raise my head off the pillow. With chin pointed toward my chest and eyes closed, a question pounds in my head: *Why me?*

*Why me with distant spread lymphoma and the Effed-up marrow?* It might be considered so unfair. All my healthful habits. No risk factors. Barely fifty-five. I'm productive, pay taxes, and vote. I try to be cheerful and remember birthdays.

*What did I do to deserve this?*

Nothing is the answer. Shit happens. There might not be a why. The universe may simply be indifferent, chaotic, random. In one sense, the *Why me?* question has a lucid, direct, and egalitarian response: *Why not me?* But this answer/question makes me angry, feel helpless, and more isolated than ever. And while we're at it, *Why me with the distant, hypochondriacal mother obsessed with her own disappointment and resentment? The weak, alcoholic father who abandoned us for a gummy blond with a fat six-year-old daughter? Why not me?*

Today, the entire pharmaceutical weight of Course B has crashed down on me. *Can't this all just be* over? *I'm useless. No good to anyone. Put me on the scrap heap.* My joints and muscles ache; my fever spikes to 102. I'm a chemical sponge and a compilation of dicey vitals and lab values that are monitored on a computer screen. I pee in a hat.

A nurse brings in morphine. Minutes later, so much better. Again. Such magic in drugs.

In my fuzzy morphine cocoon, I decide that questions such as *Why me?* and *Why not me?* are meaningless. I've been dealt a hand, a month ago in my doctor's office and decades ago in the family into which I was born. It's useless to dwell on philosophical questions that have no reliable answers. I might be the center of my universe, but it is a microscopic destination indeed.

All I can come up with after my philosophical meanderings is this: *Smile. Thank everyone. Tip big.*

There is wisdom in that line of thinking.

# Chapter 28 - Meera

AFTER I'VE FINISHED MY first Course B and have been released from the hospital, I'm back in Dr. Greyz's office and she warns me, "Your counts are so low, you could still have a heart attack and you are a big candidate for sepsis."

"Blood poisoning?"

"Yes. But your blood pressure and temperature are normal. I think you are ready for Stanford."

I sigh, from fear of the next step and exhaustion from the last.

"Have you talked to your brothers about donating stem cells?"

"Yes. They're all in," I say.

"I am happy to hear that."

The next morning, it pours. Car tires whine on water-slicked streets. With Dan at the wheel, I resume my usual role as trusty navigator. After more than two hours of stop-and-go driving through Bay Area morning commute traffic, we reach the Stanford Medical Center in Palo Alto.

We park and Dan holds my hand as we pick our way through oily puddles toward the sleek, modern building. The words Advanced Cancer Center over the main entrance tighten my stomach.

"Jesus, what are we doing? I don't belong here."

Dan tries to smile. "Pretty bleak, isn't it?"

A man slows as he hobbles toward us. Gazing at the telltale blue wool cap pulled over my ears, he smiles lopsided, and slurs, "Don't worry. You'll be fine." About my age, he is skeletal and the left side of his lower face and jaw are missing.

"Thank you," I say, trying to make my trembling lips smile back at him, forcing myself not to burst into sobs, and thinking what a radiant hero he is—attempting to make *me* feel better. All I've lost so far is my hair.

We enter the colossal building. Through a huge skylight, three stories above us, light pours into this vast white space. Voices are hushed, reverent. It feels like a temple or a spaceship. Caregivers push patients in wheelchairs. So many languages. Emaciated young people—with bald heads and bags of what I assume to be chemo hanging from their sides—shuffle by. Someone is always worse off. Help them first. Please.

Outside the floor-to-ceiling windows is a tangle of semi-tropical plants. There is a feeling of the outdoors being inside. I love that. A harpist plays *Here Comes the Sun* reminding me that George was my favorite. How I cried when he died of lung cancer.

Eighteen vials of blood are drawn from my VAP. Dr. Greyz has scheduled an all-day appointment to begin my participation as a *potential* bone marrow transplant (BMT) candidate. Meetings go on all morning; the information overwhelms me. I feel that I must burst to the surface and take a huge breath of air.

The afternoon Transplant Orientation Class is held in a nondescript, windowless conference room. Spaces like these should only contain robots. There's no moving air or changing light. These rooms are so monumentally neutral, they numb the mind. How to think or feel in such a place?

Beside Dan and me, there are four other BMT patients and their caregivers. Most of us look to be in our fifties, or younger, and many appear dazed. I am drawn to a Hindu woman in a yellow sari who wears gold bangles on her wrists. I smile, we introduce ourselves, and shake with four hands. About forty, Meera likely has the best posture I've ever seen. She seems to stand up to her disease literally and figuratively. She radiates hope. I straighten in my chair.

In sharp contrast to the lackluster room, the middle-aged, nurse-cheerleader leading the class is festive and upbeat.

"So, tell us about yourselves," she beams.

Meera begins, "I have chronic lymphocytic leukemia and will receive a stem cell transplant from my brother." She smiles revealing attractive, small white teeth. "He lives in Australia and is a perfect match."

The nurse clasps her hands to her heart and says, "Oh, that's wonderful."

After introductions, the nurse gives us more information that, in all honesty, I don't remember a word of. Maybe Dan was following; maybe all this is written down somewhere.

After the orientation, Meera and I stay to chat. She and her husband, Arjun, have a twelve-year-old daughter, Stephanie. Meera's been receiving chemo for over a year but can't hold onto a remission long enough to be transplanted. Fortunately, she has enough good days to keep her job as a high school math teacher while the chemo continues. I assure her she will reach a lasting remission.

"Do you work?" Meera asks.

"Yes. I have a home office and can get most everything done on the phone or email."

"Lucky. What do you do?"

"I direct a nationwide speakers' bureau and develop program content for physicians' education."

"Really? Well, aren't you Miss Smarty Pants?"

We both laugh. "Hardly," I say, "but I work with people who are."

"Do you have siblings?" Meera asks.

"Yes, two brothers."

"Oh, that's good. I only have one, but that's all I need. You'll be lucky too."

I smile and hug Meera whose body is birdlike.

"Best of luck to you, Meera, and get that brother over here."

"I will. And best of luck to you too. Goodbye." She waves and her bangles jingle.

Meera is a sunny interlude in this somber afternoon. Still, the day leaves me exhausted and all I want to do is collapse into bed.

Back in the car, I say to Dan, "I feel bad about saying that I only have two brothers, but Johnny might as well be in Australia too for all I know."

"I'd like to meet him someday."

I take in a deep breath then say, "It's all about sex."

"That's a jump. What do you mean?"

"Beverly is, was, Catholic. To her, sex meant babies. After Randy was born and she came down with hepatitis, her doctors told her not to have more kids. In her mind, this might have been a Get-Out-of-Sex-Free Card. My dad would have been thirty-four. Did she really think that a thirty-four-year-old, married man would be okay with throwing in the towel sexually? 'Oh, I got a doctor's note. I can't have sex anymore.' Please."

"That would've been tough on your dad."

I feel a click of guilt as Dan has also expressed a degree of frustration with our sex life. "Had she heard of a diaphragm? If this is the trip she was playing, no wonder he was frustrated. Alcoholic, no. Angry, yes."

Dan sighs. "I still don't get it."

"I believe that my father forced himself on my mother. I don't know how to say it, but it wasn't consensual. Johnny was the result, and he paid the price."

"Jesus. I'm sorry. That's so Effed up."

"Johnny was physically and emotionally abused by Beverly until he left home at eighteen, right before high school graduation. It's not a surprise that he needed to forget everything and everyone and just disappear."

I glance at the passing cars on the freeway and think about the disfigured man in the parking lot who nearly made me sob, reminding me of Johnny and how my little brother suffered. But the brave man with a partial face was strong in spite of his trauma, his anguish. He could look out of his mangled face and smile. Some cuts make us more forceful, more resilient; some ruin us. I wonder if Johnny is happy.

*Take away my hair. Take away my father. Take away my stunningly, overwhelmingly ordinary life. I will not be ruined. I will not be unhappy.*

# Chapter 29 - "At Least the Drugs Are Good"

WHILE DAN DRIVES US HOME from Stanford, I check my cell phone and see four missed voice messages from Dr. Rivers, the oncologist standing in for Dr. Greyz. I call him back.

"I got the results of your blood work from Stanford this morning. Your white count has dropped to 0.3, a critically low value."

"What do I do?"

"Watch for signs of infection, especially fever. If your temperature goes over 102, I want you in the hospital, immediately."

After I say goodbye, Dan asks, "What was that all about?"

"My white cell count is low. He wants me back in the hospital if my temp goes over 102. I'm not worried."

The next morning, Dan gives my stomach area a rest and injects Neupogen into the back of my right arm. Weak, achy, and exhausted, I spend the day in bed.

That night, so as not to wake Dan, I feel my way into our bathroom and close the door. I flip on the light and am shocked at how pale my face is, how sunken my eyes appear. Who is this woman with her expression of alarm and confusion? A violet-colored bruise, the size of my palm, blooms on my upper right arm. I wince as my hand moves over it. Fingers shaking, I unscrew the clear plastic holder of the thermometer and place the cold, hard glass under my tongue. 99.6 degrees. My sleep is fitful for the next few hours.

"You don't look so good," says Dan in the morning.

"I feel like crap. Check this out."

I fold back the sleeve of my tee shirt.

"That's where I gave you the Neupogen."

"Yeah."

"Jesus. I'm sorry."

"I'm sure it has nothing to do with you. I just need to sleep."

By 9 AM, my upper arm throbs; my temperature is 100.8.

Mid-morning, the chills come, my teeth chatter. I swallow Advil. Dan takes my temperature; it's 101.5. Then 102. I pull the down comforter around my neck and close my eyes.

Twenty minutes later it's 102.4.

"We're going to the hospital," Dan says.

"Just let me sleep. Please don't take me."

"We're going."

He wraps the light down quilt around my shoulders and bundles me into the car. One moment sweltering, the next freezing, I can't make the quilt cooperate. *Why can't I pull it around me?* He calls the ER while he drives to the hospital.

At the entrance to the ER, an orderly assists me into a wheelchair. Dan parks. We are taken into a small exam room. A nurse addresses all questions to Dan. Unable to speak, I only shake. My ears buzz. I think I might be slipping out of the wheelchair. *Have I been here a while, or only a minute?*

Dan is in front of me, lifting me back into the chair.

The nurse says something about a treatment room, now. I'm wheeled through a corridor. The lights are so bright that I close my eyes, my chin rests on my chest. I feel as if I could float away. I'm sliding out of the chair again; he pulls me back. In a small room, Dan hoists me into a hospital bed as several people rush in. *Where did he go? He must be here somewhere.*

An IV goes into my hand. A thermometer in my mouth. "Temp's 104." A Huber is pushed into my chest.

"Her right arm's bad," says Dan.

*Maybe he's behind me.*

A doctor pushes up my sleeve. Something about a blood culture. Quick. And fluids and morphine.

The manic activity of the staff slows down. The buzzing in my ears dims. With the morphine, I become woozy, even content. Dan is at my side.

I smile at him. "What a mess. At least the drugs are good."

Dan tries to smile. He looks scared. "Oh, Honey."

A nurse hands me a paper cup of ice chips. These cold, watery pebbles might be the best thing I've ever put in my mouth. I think the pain is gone. I can't find it. Dan holds my hand as I close my eyes and am now comfortable. I might sleep. I don't know. When I open my eyes, he's watching me. His expression is an odd mixture of terror and affection. I've never seen anything like it before. It's as if he's saying, *Come back to me.* He still holds my hand and offers me more ice.

Sometime later, the front desk receptionist pokes her head in and asks if we mind a visitor. Dan and I look at each other, shake our heads, and say, "Okay. Sure."

In walks our accountant, Jim, carrying an enormous basket of chocolates. My words are morphine-slurred, "How did you know we were here?"

Gesturing to the chocolates, he says, "I came to drop these off at your house and when you weren't there, I just guessed."

I reach for more ice before pulling the pink knit cap off of my hot head. There is something Fellini-esque about this whole afternoon, but the fluids and the morphine have brought me back into my body and mind.

"Well, okay."

"So, how are you?" Jim asks.

"Pretty good. At the moment."

"You look good."

I laugh, "Ha. You're the one on drugs."

"That's funny. But seriously, I thought I should check in." He nods. "Getting near the end of the year and taxes and all."

"Yes."

"Just a gentle reminder."

Dan reaches for and unwraps a Ghirardelli bar. I have always been the one in charge of all matters tax and with his attention now turned to the chocolate, I can sense him tuning out of the conversation. Jim only addresses me.

"We need to maximize your deductions before the end of the year."

"Yes."

"Exactly. And don't forget to make all of those charity contributions."

"Sure."

"Do you need to buy any office furniture?"

"I don't think so." I crunch ice between my molars.

"Sorry to burden you with this now, but it's my job to help you keep your money."

"Thanks."

"Well, I'm not going to tire you out." He stands to leave. "Now you get better. And enjoy the chocolate. I'll be in touch."

After goodbyes, I look at Dan, shake my head, and say, "How did *that* happen?"

"Weird, huh?"

"How did he know we were here?"

"Beats me."

"Maybe he can use his powers of ESP to do our taxes without my help."

"Don't worry about it, Honey. It'll get taken care of."

I pop an ice chip and question just how *that* might happen.

"Do you think Jim wonders how long he'll be my accountant?"

"Stop it."

"It's a joke."

"Not funny."

Back upstairs, in room 522, again, the lights are turned off. *Do they keep this room reserved for me?* Draperies are drawn. The teeth-chattering chills begin once more. I beg for blankets. Dan pulls them around my face and body, but still I shake. Then I am burning up, throwing off the blankets, and reaching for ice. The room is sweltering, or, no, maybe it's freezing.

"Please make the racket go away," I moan, pushing my palms to my temples.

"Honey,"—he strokes the side of my face—"there's no racket."

Through unfocussed eyes, I watch Dan watching me. "Please. Make it go away," I say.

His face is stricken. "I love you."

"I love you too."

Every couple of hours, I get more morphine. Before dawn, Dan lies in a recliner beside me. I ache. Sweating, I sit up and peer into the corners of the shadowy room, watching my husband sleep.

The last time I saw my father he lay in a mortuary and slept as well— the long, dreamless sleep from which no one wakes. He'd died two evenings before of a heart attack. So sudden, he never got to say I love you, or goodbye, or thank you to anyone. Through these last tormented hours, at least I'd been able to tell my husband I love him.

The July evening my dad died was hot, cloudless, and without a breeze. He'd come home from his engineering firm and after dinner, as he'd done so many times before, watered his backyard garden. Idel found him. Perhaps she'd heard a strange sound or just noticed him gone. Maybe the hose was still running. I never asked. These were intimate details, and I didn't think she would want me probing into the private moments surrounding my father's death. The paramedics tried to resuscitate him.

*Was his death painful or so quick he didn't notice? Did he call someone's name? Who did he think of? Was it me? My mother? My brothers? What was the last thing he felt? Remorse? Fear? Peace? Nothing?*

Putting my hands to my throbbing temples, I sense a frequency, a tone. What am I hearing? Is death a sound? Does it just slip in and separate the life from the body? I fear that death might be that simple, that quick, that incontestable. Did my father hear this tone in his garden on the evening he died?

My hands sweep over the humid sheet. The feel of damp, of warmth, of soft cotton calms me. My husband's steady breathing calms me. Even the pain in my arm calms me. I know I am still here, in my body.

WEEKS AFTER MY FATHER DIED, I called Idel and asked about his will—as delicately as I could; these questions are rarely delicate.

"He died intestate."

I wasn't sure of the word intestate. It sounded almost medical and confused me.

"He gave his shotgun to his nephew. That's all he owned."

*Oh, except for his engineering firm with dozens of employees.*

"What about the business?"

"That's mine. That was never your dad's."

*What?* He'd started the firm and worked there for more than twenty years. He was so infuriatingly passive. Why didn't he ever stand up for his kids? The bitterness of his abandonment burned within me all over again.

Seems that Idel demanded the business as her payment for years of writing alimony and child support checks. For working full time. I get that Idel would feel owed. But she married a man with four children. What did she think was going to happen? That his kids and ex-wife would just disappear? I know she certainly hoped so.

During that conversation, Idel told me that if my dad hadn't died, they would have divorced. It was in the works. It often seemed that they could barely stand to be in the same room together. The meanness between them was a noxious smell in the air. How would my relationship with my dad have changed had he been divorced from Idel and away from the stifling Stacy? It was a question that I would ask myself a thousand times without an answer.

# Chapter 30 - I Made It to Halloween

THE DOOR TO MY HOSPITAL room swings open and Big Bird bounces in.

"Happy Halloween," says Dr. Arent.

I blink then squint at the lightly bearded, handsome face surrounded by bright yellow feathers. He bird-hops to my bed. "How are you?"

My reply is something between a whimper and a hum, accompanied by a weak smile.

"Anything hurt?"

I pull my arm out from under the blanket. During the night, it began to swell and the Neupogen injection site is as purple as an eggplant and throbbing. He rotates my arm to get a better look and gently places his hand on the darkened area.

"It's hot."

"Yeah."

He touches my shoulder, "We're going to get you through this. I promise. I'm ordering an additional antibiotic."

I nod.

"Buzz for morphine when you need it." Big Bird hops out of the room.

Dr. Arent is such a good doctor. I wonder what he knows about the moment of death. He must have seen it many times. I've seen dead people, but never watched the life leave someone.

It might be much easier than I imagine. I want to ask him but don't have the strength. At least I'm alive. I've made it to Halloween.

Dan comes into the room with coffee from the espresso cart and sits on my bed. I put my head on his chest and listen to his strong, regular heartbeat. The same life-giving thump that had stopped pulsing through my father's body. With my face turned toward his neck, I breathe in the smell of soap, something honeyed like cardamom, and a trace of salt. The scent of a living body. My father's scent, which I knew so well as a child—aftershave, cigarette smoke, and alcohol—I couldn't describe in the years after he stopped drinking and smoking.

The call about my father's death came from Stacy on a Wednesday night; I shuddered in Dan's arms. A wave of grief made me wobble and I held onto my husband who supported me as I was engulfed by the emotional deluge of the death of a parent. Beyond the waves of grief at his passing—that submerged me under a murky blue pain—I felt so cheated. Grief battled resentment in the aching emotional tug-of-war the night my dad died. He'd left me again. I was thirty-six; my dad sixty.

We'd seen each other three days before. Uncharacteristically distant and fatigued, he seemed frail and had little to say. Was he thinking of things more profound than my casual recounting of Dan's latest business trip or the new tile we'd ordered for our bathroom? Did he have a premonition about his death in seventy-two hours? And, if my father had suspected, felt a foreboding, might he have taken me aside that last Sunday? Taken me aside and said what? What does a man thinking he is facing death say to his grown daughter with whom he has shared so little? And, had his death been anticipated, had *I* had a warning, what would *I* have said to *him?* Would I have been less than kind? Told him I loved him, but that he failed us all? He'd made a huge, painful mess that we all had to live with while he got out and barely looked back. At least, that's what it felt like. Did his failures, weaknesses, his inability to express love haunt him the rest of his life? I'd imagine they might.

And what will be my burden? My regret? Who or what will I think of in the instant of my death? How will I feel in that moment when we legendarily see our lives pass before our eyes?

I alternate between freezing and burning up. The nurses inject more morphine, more antibiotics into my IV. In my feverish dream state, I can't leave the questions alone. *Did my father sense his death? Will I sense mine? Does death have the same shape, and sound, and smell for everyone?*

Or does it depend? Was the place of my father's last consciousness his garden? Or could he still see himself a day later in the mortuary with its consuming hush, deep carpets, and somber tones? The place where he and I shared our final hour—the mortuary décor reflecting what mourners were expected to do with their emotions: to subdue and swallow them, to remain quiet, numb, and well mannered.

A funeral director escorted Dan, Idel, and me from the lobby to an anteroom with a gleaming beige linoleum floor, shaded windows, and a double sliding door on the opposite wall. Was this the entry to where morticians did what they did with care and compassion? Picturing my father behind those doors, where he had been embalmed, made me panic. He lay on a gurney. Wearing a navy-blue woolen shirt, a thin white cotton bedspread was tucked snugly around his mid chest. We pulled three folding chairs around the gurney; Dan and I on one side, Idel on the other. She was reserved and did not cry; she touched her husband once on the shoulder but did not say his name.

After some minutes of silence, Dan thoughtfully asked if I would like to be alone with him. So grateful for his question, I wouldn't have had the courage to request that Idel leave me alone with my father. And without understanding it, that was exactly what I wanted.

They left and I touched my father's cool face. The embalming fluids had made it hard and waxy. His broad shoulders and neatly combed goatee gave him a regal quality. Expanded, his chest appeared as if he had just taken in a deep breath. As I kissed him, I knew I would never forget the sensation of his wooden cheek on my lips. I placed the side of my face on his rough shirt. I had no tears, just an immense longing. Closing my eyes, I breathed in the scents of wool and formaldehyde, like the scent of decaying flowers. We'd had so little time, just the two of us, that it struck me as a cruel joke that when we were finally alone together in the same room, he was not there.

Tom, Randy, and Diane flew up for the memorial service. Since none of us had any idea how to contact Johnny, it would be many years until he knew our father had died.

IT'S BEEN OVER TWENTY-FOUR HOURS since I was admitted to the hospital and Dan is still with me. My fever now hovers around 101. The antibiotics have started to win the sepsis battle.

"You need to go home," I tell him.

Bleary-eyed and exhausted, Dan reluctantly agrees. "I'll be checking in with the nurses."

My sleep is fitful, drug induced. Waking in the morning, the all-over body aches are less intense, but my right arm throbs non-stop. Double its size, the swelling starts at my fingers and continues up my arm to my shoulders and around my upper back. I can't lift it higher than my waist.

# Chapter 31 - My Bologna Arm and a Football Game

THE NEXT DAY, I AM SENT home with my aching bologna arm and a ten-day course of Septra double strength b.i.d. (oral, twice a day). Diagnosis: *sepsis, a whole-body, blood inflammation caused by severe infection.* Fatal in one of four cases.

A week later, Elspeth is home again and convinces Dan and me to go to the Cal-USC football game with her. Wanting to spend as much time together as possible, I agree. Being a student at USC, Elspeth roots for the red and gold Trojans while Dan and I, both Cal Berkeley grads, don't much care. If our university loyalties lie with U.C. Berkeley, our checkbook is a USC captive.

Tens of thousands of fans cram into the California Memorial Stadium. How I manage—with my bulging arm pounding with pain, my lightheadedness, and weakness—I don't know. Sheer willpower gets me up the stairs to our seats. Although the roar of the crowd is earsplitting, I somehow survive all four quarters but cannot tell you which side won. Elspeth has taken off with a few friends. Walking the long blocks back to our car, supported by Dan, I force myself not to faint or throw up, or both. Dan opens the door for me and I collapse into the passenger seat. At home, he helps me undress and I fall into bed.

In my sleep, I'd tossed off the fleece blanket and lie on my back under only a sheet. It is 1:20 AM. With the back of my hand, I brush the damp skin between my breasts. Except for Dan's steady breathing, the room is quiet and dark. Illness and despair are pounding weights on my chest.

My fingertips graze the infected area in my upper right arm. The pain is sharp and immediate; I let out a low moan. I'm thirsty and want to get up. Then I notice a warmth next to the bed, and I extend my right hand over the carpeted floor; my hand feels pleasantly relaxed, as if being lightly supported. I look. Around my side of the bed, rising about two feet off the carpet, is a pink mist.

Am I dreaming, hallucinating, or having a drug reaction?

No. My eyes are open. While tempted to touch it, I don't; it might disappear. With my right hand still extended over the mist, the pressure lifts from my chest. My limbs relax. It can't be there. But it is—pink and warm and hovering around my bed.

Some people are born with faith, like curly hair. Some find it, like first love after seventy. For others, akin to travel to Greenland, it never happens. The truly faithful have taken simple hope one giant step forward, as in a spiritual Mother-May-I game, in which you get to move from simply wanting or hoping for something to happen to believing and knowing that it will. Handshake with the cosmos. Deal done.

Perhaps the mist is a free transfer—from illness to health—a Get-Out-of-Cancer Ticket already punched. All of us can hope; even non-believers can hope.

1:45 AM, I close my eyes and am peaceful. Everything will be okay. I sleep.

The next morning the pink mist is gone. I don't tell anyone and would feel odd talking about it. Like I felt funny telling Elspeth about the hallucinogenic way trees, hills, the sky, and colors quivered and seemed to enfold me in a blissful embrace. Is this the peace that Johnny sought with psilocybin and LSD? The question occurs: *Was the mist a glimpse into death?* That possibility is not frightening. I am serene. The mist does not reappear.

TEN DAYS LATER, THE BUGS in my bloodstream are gone, but the infection in my arm remains a continual misery. From the back of my neck to my fingertips, my arm remains swollen twice its size. It's difficult to bend, difficult to write or do much of anything else, and does not look as if it even belongs on my body.

The area where the Neupogen had been injected two weeks earlier is hot, blue-black, and hurts like hell. On my last dose of Septra, the aching becomes so intense that I down a Vicodin. It helps a little, but the Vicodin and Septra combo messes up my stomach. All day, I'm on the verge of vomiting.

Besides the continual pain and swelling, I'm losing hope that this infection will ever go away. My gloom is affecting my marriage. Dan and I are becoming emotionally frayed. We sometimes don't know what to say to each other, or even where to look. It's not blame but a testy resentment that can settle in between us. I understand that annoyance and have felt a pinch of it from him. It would have been the same had the tables been turned. Who wants their lives capsized by cancer? No one, and neither of us are saints.

So willing to help in so many ways, cooking is not one of them. Dan's pique comes out as carelessness. How can someone make so much noise cooking a simple meal? There is bedlam between the pots and pans. The microwave door slams shut. Since beginning chemo, sounds have become amplified and the din is nearly unbearable. We try to be pleasant, but sometimes I am less than polite when I ask him to please reduce the ruckus. He grumbles over so much work. Who can blame him? Everything is on his shoulders. He carries such a heavy load.

Thank God for food from friends, so he doesn't have to cook every night.

We watch the news. People in New Orleans are still displaced from Hurricane Katrina. They have no kitchens. Many have no home to go back to. They are sleeping in the Superdome. Kind souls in kayaks and canoes rescue neighbors and their pets. I feel I shouldn't complain, then feel entitled to. Would I trade places with the poor, uprooted people in New Orleans? What a stupid question. No, of course not.

The bigger deal than the infection or the pain in my arm is delaying—now for a couple of weeks—the start of my third cycle of Hyper-CVAD. I can't have any treatment that will suppress my already paltry number of white cells, or the infection will get worse.

*Just shoot me if it does.*

The homeless people of New Orleans wait for the water to recede; I wait for the infection to do the same.

# Chapter 32 - He Could Operate on King Kong

THE NEXT MORNING, I CAN'T THINK of anything but the pain in my arm. I call the infectious disease department at Kaiser and plead to be seen. Because I can't grasp the steering wheel with my right hand, Laurie, my cheerful helper, loving and level-headed, drives me to the afternoon appointment. The physician asks how long I've had the infection, what meds I'm taking, and the level of pain. I pride myself on being an easy patient, of not asking for much, and doing whatever I can for myself. Today, I am the same: cooperative, reasonable, and friendly, answering all questions politely with measure and precision.

"Well, nothing else can be done, pharmaceutically. Lancing is your only option."

"Lancing?"

"The infection must be expelled from your arm."

"How is that done?" I ask.

"With a scalpel and a local." She looks at me as if I am a sniveling three-year-old.

"Would it be possible to have a wee bit of Valium to take the edge off?"

I think the doctor might find the *wee bit* part humorous and be more inclined to go along with the request.

"No." Her response is fast and emphatic, giving me no room for hope.

"So, is there another way to make this nasty business a little less so?"

"Your other option is a full-on surgery in the OR with a general anesthesia."

"There's no middle ground?"

"You must compose yourself."

Immediately insulted, I am speechless and want to blurt out, "You are a bloodless bitch."

The cruel comment shocks me. Why would a doctor say such a thing? I am the one carrying around this throbbing bologna arm that hurts so much it makes my teeth ache. I am the one being pickled in chemo for a life-threatening cancer. I am the one who nearly expired from sepsis. What a vile, thoughtless hag. A little compassion, please.

"I … I am composed. I'm just exploring my options."

"I'll call and make an appointment. They should be able to take you this afternoon."

I fight against the threatening tears and imagine the dragon doctor gloating that I will suffer.

I hate her.

From my medical record of the visit: *Patient was emotionally upset otherwise non-toxic.* [???]

Non-toxic? Yes, *I* was non-toxic. *The doctor* was the one who was freaking toxic.

Laurie and I take the elevator down to the surgical offices. Expecting a kindly Dr. Welby type, I am nonplussed when shown into the office of a huge, ruddy, and oily surgeon. His hairy hands are massive. He could operate on King Kong without anesthesia. My palms are damp. There is pressure on my chest, and my breath comes from my throat.

Laurie offered and I ask if she can come in with me. *No*—another fast, emphatic response. A sweet, young nurse shows me into a small procedure room and asks me to lie down on my stomach so the super-sized scalpel wielder has access to the back of my right arm. When he injects the lidocaine into the infection, I nearly jump off the table. It feels like a stab with a sizzling knife.

"Hold still," he grumbles.

Clutching the nurse's hand, I will myself to be quiet and motionless. When he inserts the scalpel into the wound, I'm afraid I might be sick. Moans escape my lips.

"I've made the incision and pus is just pouring out of your arm."

I can't tell if he's proud of himself or disgusted.

"Great," I mumble with a mixture of relief and distaste.

Then he starts pushing on the incision and I wince and moan again. It feels as though his entire and considerable weight is pressing down on my aching, bloated arm. Determined to get through it, I do not allow myself to beg him to stop. After prolonged minutes of pain, he says, "Now, your job is to keep it open and flowing."

I grimace.

"That means twice a day you must run gallons of hot, hot water on it and then have someone press out as much pus as you can stand." He sounds impatient.

From my medical record: *Husband helping to milk b.i.d.*

"How long do we have to do that?"

"Only a couple of days. Then it will start to heal."

Walking back to the car, I hang onto Laurie. My legs wobble. I am weak, and beat up (again), but hopeful that the worst is behind me. I tell Dan about the expressing to eliminate the infection. Fortunately, he is no milquetoast and when tasked with helping—however unpleasant the chore—he takes it on with commitment. So, twice a day as I lean over the kitchen sink, he sprays the hottest water on my arm that I can tolerate. Then he presses on the incision producing pus and other noxious fluids that wash down the drain. By the end of each of these sessions, I am shaking and begging him to stop. But this infection will not be defeated and the damned gunk just keeps coming. Expression goes on twice a day for seven days; it seems it will never stop. On the morning of the eighth day, we are busy and can't go through the b.i.d. torture. That night he nearly scalds my arm, but no matter how hard he presses, he can't get the incision to open up.

The following week, the surgical tissue cultures come back and verify that the arm infection was the same as that in my bloodstream: *RARE GROWTH ESCMYICHIA COLI.* My arm begins to heal. My white cell counts are back up to where I can begin the Hyper-CVAD regimen again and have those cells knocked down to the substrata without the threat of the arm becoming reinfected. Hallelujah. *Sort of.*

# Chapter 33 - Straight from the Chinese Hamster Ovary

WHAT BADASS WOULD SAY, "Hey, I'll bet the Chinese hamster ovary might offer a cure for cancer?" Some genius, or mad scientist? But that little hormone-producing rodent gland is exactly where Rituxan®, the next step in my treatment, comes from.

Like every other drug, Rituxan has a laundry list of side effects. The one that frightens me most: Serious infections that *can happen during and after treatment and can lead to death.* Great, just great.

A 50-mm test tube of science: Rituxan and chemotherapy work differently. Chemo targets and kills cells that are dividing. As adults, much of our cell division has already occurred, and many of our cells only divide into new cells to repair damage or grow hair or nails. In cancer, cells divide to single-mindedly increase their population. They keep dividing and multiplying (clever little mathematicians) until they form a mass that becomes a lump—a tumor. Due to this frenzied division, cancer cells are more likely to be targeted and killed by chemotherapy than healthy cells.

Rituxan does not distinguish between healthy and cancerous B cells (B cells are where Mantle Cell Lymphoma arises); it kills them all. This presents a conundrum. Chemo kills malignant B cells. Rituxan kills even healthy B cells, just the ones I might need to fight another life-threatening infection. Yet in clinical trials, addition of Rituxan to chemotherapy produced better outcomes and led to more cancer patients achieving remission. Dr. Greyz convinces me to take the risk.

Because Rituxan is less toxic than Hyper-CVAD, I can receive it as an outpatient in an infusion clinic. In the large, oblong room, patients and visitors chat, laugh, and cough. Someone is eating French fries. The monitors—signaling that medication bottles are empty, or the infusion rate needs to be increased—beep off and on. Shoes squeak across the turquoise-and-gray linoleum squares. Plastic dividers, like shower curtains, between infusion chairs rustle open and closed. The lights are dimmable. Some people sleep. How can they with all the noise? I can choose to recline or remain upright in my blue fake leather chair. I sit upright and work on my laptop. Compared to chemo, this is a breeze.

While receiving this first of many, multi-hour drips of Rituxan, Randy and his family arrive at the infusion clinic. Seeing my bald head, hollow body, and a bottle of medication dripping into me through a tube and needle in my chest must be a shock. *Should I apologize, be embarrassed, or try to make a joke?* I smile.

"Hi. You found me."

How could I have prepared them for this? I couldn't. No one cries, neither do they rush toward me. Subdued and cautious, Randy and Diane kiss me softly on either side of my face. I air kiss them back. My niece and nephew, remaining in the doorway, wave and try to smile. The fear, pain, and confusion on their faces grieves me. I want to tell them that it's okay, that this is really progress, even if it looks like a scene out of *A Clockwork Orange*.

Dan buys a pre-made Thanksgiving dinner from a local supermarket. To me, the food still has that woody, chemical taste. I drink more wine than I should to dilute a melancholy that scares the crap out of me. Battling a paralyzing inertia, my need to curl into a fetal position and pull a blanket over my head is nearly irresistible; but I force myself to get out of bed, to speak, and eat a little. We've received our new furniture, so at least my family can sit down. We take smiling, silly pictures. People make rabbit ears over each other's heads. But when the camera isn't clicking, all of us look older.

On the evening before they leave, I ask Randy if he's seen Johnny.

"No. Yes."

"What?"

"The last time I saw him we didn't say anything."

"What?' I ask again.

I passed him on the beach, but we both just walked on by."

This scene is painfully easy for me to visualize. They were never close as kids.

"Had something happened, between the two of you?"

"Yeah. Years ago, I found out where he lived and went to talk to him about what he was doing with his life."

"What did he say?"

"Beyond selling drugs, taking it easy and surfing."

I shudder, not from shock but from the recognition of what I'd always feared. "I'd hoped that drug dealing wasn't going to be the path he chose."

"I thought I might be able to turn him around, but clearly it wasn't going to happen. He operates in a drug underground."

My jaw tightens. "There are reasons for that."

"I know you blame Mom for how he turned out, but he's old enough to make his own decisions."

Randy was too young to see or remember the damage inflicted on Johnny, but I do not want to argue with him. I'm only sad. It's tragic when children are raised in an environment so toxic that—years later, as adults—they don't even say hello when they walk past each other. Of the four of us kids, Johnny and I had it the hardest. For us, it came down to self-defense. He'd been kicked out, and I escaped into the world to make my way. It was each of us against everything and everyone else. Struggling. Wounded. Alone without siblings or parents. So strange in a family that had once numbered six.

"I have no idea where he is now. Our last conversation was almost thirty years ago."

"At least you tried to help. That's more than I ever did," I say.

"Don't count on seeing him again. He's a goner."

I fight off a pang of guilt for not doing more—something—for my brilliant little brother.

"But Tom or I, maybe both of us, will be a match for you. Don't worry. We've got this."

"I know you do," I say.

The next morning, Randy and his family return home. I continue to force myself to get out of bed. Food tastes like rancid cardboard. I drink to drown. With luck, I think, someday we will all look young in the silly rabbit-eared photographs.

I am readmitted for a third round of chemo and my fifth hospitalization since September. I should be on round four, but we lost nearly a month fighting the arm infection and septicemia. It's been a week since Dan attempted the last expression, but my arm remains swollen, red, and tender, as if a lingering contamination still festers in the muscle. When Dr. Greyz visits me this morning in room 522, I tell her that I am drowning in another person's life.

# Chapter 34 - Rescue Me, Please

DR. FOWLER—THE PSYCHIATRIST SENT by Dr. Greyz—doesn't intend to poison me. A sympathetic man, rotund, and likely in his seventies, he visits me before breakfast. He spends a lot of time asking about my early life, which I am convinced is entirely unrelated to the chemical, drug-induced darkness that immobilizes me and out of which I cannot escape. He reviews my meds and focuses on dexamethasone, the steroid I've been taking since chemo began.

Yes, he tells me, dexamethasone is the essential 'D' part of the Hyper-CVAD cocktail, but its benefits come with a steep price tag. Pick just about any side effect and it will be associated with dexamethasone—but those affecting the psyche are the ones torturing me: depression, emotional instability, insomnia, and mood swings.

Dr. Fowler says that I am one of the unlucky ten percent of patients who experience severely debilitating psychological side effects and that my crushing depression over Thanksgiving was likely due to a too-rapid *withdrawal* of the steroid.

Now back on 40 mg of dexamethasone daily—considered a decent-sized dose—he recommends tapering off the steroid when this chemo round ends, as well as a "rescue" drug. Thank God. I am hopeful that this taper can now counteract, or even prevent, another emotional shattering.

After Dr. Fowler leaves, I receive my morning meds. The 40 mg of dexamethasone kicks in. I buy a latte. My energy comes roaring back. Still on the steroid rollercoaster, I make bubbly phone calls. In my medicinal-caffeine high, the sense of hopelessness subsides, until mid-afternoon when my little amusement park ride takes a dip and plunges me into a deep, depressive hole.

Throughout the night, staff hang new bags of chemo and other meds. Having a major case of insomnia—a steroid side effect—I get two Ativans from the nurses and take two full Restorils and one-half of a Valium (both of the latter snuck in from home). Normally—well, this much is never normal—these many downers would have kept me asleep for a day and a half.

At 7:00 AM, I'm awake again, swallow another 40 mg of dexamethasone, and drink a double latte that pumps me into a chemical giddiness. I phone Dan at his office.

"I hope it won't be months before we have sex again," I say.

"Trust me. I'm not thinking about that."

"A man? Not thinking about sex?"

"Well, I think about it; but you know what I'm saying."

"I love you, and I mean it about the sex," I say.

"Me too."


AT THIRTY-SIX, DAN HADN'T been ready to settle down. I thought of him as a desperado, a *puer aeternus*, a guy with the Peter Pan syndrome, forever young. We'd had a rocky beginning. I'd broken up with him, he with me, but after a year of fits and starts, we were ready to be a couple. Besides, I'd never shared a bed with a man who recited poetry. That got me.

The night I fell in love with Dan, we'd gone to the Nutcracker ballet in San Francisco then had dinner at Max's Opera Café. Back home we made love for half the night, then he held me and began to recite *Ode to a Nightingale,* stanza after stanza.

*"My heart aches, and a drowsy numbness pains*
*My sense, as though of hemlock I had drunk,*
*Or emptied some dull opiate to the drains*
*One minute past, and Lethe-wards had sunk:*
*'Tis not through envy of thy happy lot,*

*But being too happy in thine happiness,*
*That thou, light-wingèd Dryad of the trees,*
*In some melodious plot*
*Of beechen green, and shadows numberless,*
*Singest of summer in full-throated ease."*

At six-four, Dan is a Bill Hurt look-alike who recites Keats (even though the poem is about death). Nice, huh? We were married in 1983; he was thirty-eight and I was thirty-two.

# Chapter 35 - High-End Math

DR. PORTER—ON CALL FOR DR. GREYZ—is way too sure of himself. A balding, professorial-looking oncologist—wearing a bow tie and appearing to be at least five years past retirement—he approaches the small whiteboard in my room, pulls a dry-erase marker from his pocket, and starts making calculations. He's here to prescribe the rescue medicine that Dr. Fowler recommended yesterday and to instruct me on tapering the dexamethasone. As he scribbles numbers on the board, he mumbles something about Body Mass Index—mine isn't much anymore—the half-life of dexamethasone, and some other mathematical jargon. His conclusion after this high-end math: one dexamethasone tomorrow, one the day after, and one-half on day three. To me, his plan carries a strong odor of catastrophe. How can forty milligrams—for days—then ten, ten, and five be considered a taper?

"How about thirty, twenty, ten, and five?" I ask.

He shakes his head. "No. All you need is a little in your system. Ten milligrams will adequately taper the medication."

"You think that will be enough?" I'm wary.

He waves his hand. "Plenty."

I remember another doctor who waved a dismissive hand at me and mumbled something about a virus.

After my morning meds, including 40 mg of dexamethasone, I'm released at 11:00 AM with a bottle of Seroquel, the rescue drug recommended by Dr. Fowler, and a plastic vial containing three lonely dexamethasone tablets. On the way home, I'm as restless as a rip tide.

My sleep is light again, not surprising since the damned steroid still floods my system.

I'M ON A TWO-WEEK BREAK from chemo. Feeling okay the next morning, I convince Dan to go to work. Downing my one allotted dexamethasone, I begin to organize my closet. I cannot decide if I need that extra bathrobe and do not understand why I am so annoyed about those heels I never wear. Damn heels. Why do I have to think about them at all?

The task overwhelms me, but I can't stop. I have a metallic tongue and brush and floss my teeth twice. I put clothes into Goodwill bags, then take them out. The clanging of hangers brings tears to my eyes. I shake my head to try and stop the buzzing in my ears. I rub my too-warm bald head; I should eat but can't. Maybe a cappuccino. I might be cold and think about putting on a sweater. Telling myself, *I can do this*, I pace around my bedroom and hyperventilate. I have to move. It's only some sweaters; it's only chemo and steroids. It's only cancer.

I swallow a Seroquel. Maybe I should start some laundry.

I don't know it, but Seroquel is used in the treatment of schizophrenia; acute, manic episodes associated with bipolar disorder; and for patients with major depressive disorder. I naively assume that Seroquel is a relative of Xanax, a nice little tranquilizer used for short-term relief of anxiety. Like a martini but without the carbs or calories.

By 3:30 PM, my anxiety level is at high alert. And, we've had a technology meltdown—all but one telephone is dead; only my office phone downstairs has a dial tone. Swallowing an Ativan, I call Dan. Sent straight to voice mail, I try to sound casual, saying I'm not feeling well, but tell him not to worry.

After leaving the message, I lie down on the couch in the upstairs family room. Pressing my knees to my chest—literally holding myself together—I now know what "crawling out of one's skin" means. Where is my cell phone? My downstairs office phone starts ringing and continues to ring at intervals over the next two hours. I'm sure it's Dan and tell myself to get up, but I cannot move from under a light woolen blanket.

The house gets dark and cold. Desperate, I manage to get to the bathroom and swallow another Ativan. Back on the couch in my fetal position, I wait and tremble but no pharmaceutical can touch this. Nothing brings sleep or eases the panic. I am terrified to take another Seroquel.

Finally, his key is in the lock.

"Honey? You here?"

I can only shiver.

"Honey?" He calls again and hurries upstairs.

"I'm here," I murmur.

"God, what happened?"

"You took so long."

"I should have known something was wrong. Why didn't you answer your cell phone?"

"I don't know where it is. I want wine."

"Should you be drinking?"

"I want wine."

He comes back upstairs with a half glass of white wine and a large tumbler of Wild Turkey for himself. He turns on the heater and wraps another blanket around my shoulders. With the first sip of Sauvignon Blanc, a tiny ripple of calm moves through me.

"I don't know if I can do this."

"I'm so sorry. I'll be home tomorrow. I'll help you."

"I wish you could."

Day two of the fake dexamethasone taper, I swallow my one allotted pill and go back to the closet but still cannot decide if I love or hate a new pair of tennis shoes. Maybe I should eat. Should I? By mid-afternoon, anxiety and depression bear down on my chest and squeeze my solar plexus making breathing difficult. Giving up on the Goodwill bags, I pace from room to room and try to avoid Dan so I won't have to talk. In the bathroom, the bottle of Seroquel sits on the white granite countertop. Grasping it in a shaky hand, I open it, and flush the evil pills down the toilet. Craving only oblivion, I swallow a Restoril and go to bed.

Day three, I take my half tablet. The weight on my chest is less. The poisonous crap is leaving my body, but I still cannot decide what to do with myself. I pretend to nap and spend most of the day avoiding my husband and attempting to shut off my own mind.

In the afternoon of day four, I can breathe. The weight on my chest has lifted. Dan builds a fire. I make popcorn. We drink beer and sit on the couch. I taste salt. Butter. Beer. It's as if this is the first time I've tasted any of these flavors and they fairly explode in my mouth. I can't get enough. More popcorn. More beer. Thank God this steroid has left me.

"Tomorrow I might go shopping for an area rug. For the bedroom," I say.

"Honey, maybe you should save your strength for getting well."

"I'd like to have a little fun."

In Dan's eyes there's worry and it's not just about the Visa bill.

"Is it the best thing to be out so soon after… after all this?"

"I need to do something."

"I get that. But we can't take chances or deny what's going on."

"Why can't I deny what's going on? Who says I can't?"

He raises his eyebrows. I've denied so much. It hasn't always been wise, but I'm just talking about shopping.

"When I was eleven and my dad had moved out, I was at our mailbox when a neighbor asked me if my parents were divorced. My skin went hot and prickly. We were Catholic. I was too ashamed to look at her and said, 'No, they aren't divorced.' So, she says, 'Well, I haven't seen your dad in a long time.' So I said, 'Oh, he's around.'"

"Jesus, that's a mean thing to ask a kid."

"All I could do was flat-out deny what was going on."

"I don't blame you. You're right. Go shop for your rug."

I smile, kiss my husband, and take a swig of beer.

# Chapter 36 - Clean Up That Attitude

MY DAYS AT HOME, BETWEEN cycles of chemo, resemble a couple of classic dreams I've had for years. I'm either in college or working as a waitress. Not surprising since both activities took up the majority of my twenties. If in college, it's the day of finals and I've never been to class. I'm half naked and have no idea where I'm supposed to go. If the dream is in a restaurant, I'm like a pinball being flung back and forth from one table to another—never taking an order or delivering so much as a glass of water.

I whine to my friend Gael. We've known and loved each other for forty-five years.

"I'm drowning in chaos. I can't concentrate and don't know what to do. I'm blaming myself for every bad thing that's ever happened to me."

"Hey, girl. You need an attitude adjustment. Call these folks."

The Center for Attitudinal Healing is a local organization that has been around for decades. Their vision says it all. The Center provides services to help you *"...in finding ways of healing attitudes, choosing love rather than fear, peace rather than conflict, and the peace that forgiveness can bring to each of us. Our work not only deals with illness and dying, loss and grief, but with living fully each moment and healing relationships in all parts of our lives."*

The Center's services sound like sturdy lifeboats tacking right toward me.

The Center supports two groups for which I would be a "fit": People Facing Life-Threatening Illness, and Women with Metastasized Cancer. Neither really a club one wants to join; still, I am hopeful of friendship, support, and release from negative thinking.

The Center, tucked under a towering stand of redwoods, is on a side street in the picturesque seaside town of Sausalito. It is a cold, sunny December day. From under the trees, I walk into a pool of sunshine. Eyes closed, the light and warmth sink into my shoulders and relax them. I breathe deeply and imagine my heart and mind opening to new ideas.

Inside the modest building there is no formal lobby or anyone to ask where my "class" might be. I wander down the main hallway then locate a schedule taped to the colorless, beige wall.

The classroom is bright and clean. We sit in an assortment of mismatched chairs in a loose circle. There is no facilitator, just five of us at the Women with Metastasized Cancer meeting. I feel awkward and unsure of what to do, but three of the women have been here before and know the ropes. We take turns talking, if and when we want. Everyone has a different story and each is wrenching. One woman in her thirties with advanced breast cancer has taken to drinking her own, *and* her husband's, urine. As bizarre and desperate as this might sound, the practice has a medical name: Urotherapy. While Westerners likely have a problem with the very concept, let alone trying this, drinking human urine has been part of traditional medical practices in many Asian countries for thousands of years. In fact, the woman drinking urine is Asian American. Her story shocks and saddens me, but judgments are frowned on at the Center so I just sit quietly and listen.

Another woman claims that it is nonsense to assume we will die of our cancers; a truck might hit us on our way home. True. Takeaway: *Stop thinking about dying and start thinking about living.* I nod my head but picture the semi barreling down on me.

A third woman and I share Dr. Greyz as an oncologist; but the woman complains that because of the Ukrainian accent she can't understand her, which I think is ridiculous. She also reveals that Dr. Porter (the high-end math guy who "calculated" my fake dexamethasone taper) had met with her in November and told her to "get her affairs in order." Do doctors really say that? Deeply shaken, she followed his instruction. But just weeks later, he reported to her that her clinical indicators are "looking pretty good." How he got through medical school is a wonder since he is apparently no better at prognostication than he is at arithmetic.

Trying to be open-minded, I can't help but shrink at this retelling of catastrophe. A surreal, fun-house tinge permeates the meeting. Is it even healthful to dwell on these details? And, while trying to *encourage* healing attitudes, the Center's philosophy of wellness does not *feel* healthy to me—the subtext hints that *we* just might be responsible for *our* cancers. Yes, the message is subtle; but if the Center maintains that *"Health is inner peace. Healing is letting go of fear,"* isn't there just the faintest suggestion that if we weren't all so darned keyed up, we might not have gotten sick in the first place? I hate that kind of thinking.

Okay, there's smoking and lung cancer, but to imply that negative thinking is the cause of our suffering is outrageous. Haven't we cancer patients been through enough? Do we have to look back on our lives, see how we've screwed up, and admit we are now responsible for this too? Give me a break. Nothing I did, or did not do, could have prevented Mantle Cell Lymphoma. And that's the straight, simple truth.

I do not want to talk about freaking cancer. I never go back to the Center but decide that I will try to avoid—as a Buddhist friend says—any more *stinkin' thinkin'*.

It is well into December. The days are short; the nights are long and dark. Sometimes, the thought of Christmas makes me want to weep; other times it brings me intense happiness. Lights appear on houses. While we have no tree—neither of us has the strength or motivation to put one up and a living tree might carry microbes that could send me back in the hospital with another infection—Dan strings bright white lights around our front door. Cards with Madonnas and grinning reindeer arrive. Like my head, the branches of the maples on our street are bare; in this season, the work of the tree is internal. Chemo is the same. Only the death of the old is seen; there is no visible promise yet of anything new. But perhaps by spring my head will sprout wild new growth, preparing yet again for one more glorious season.

# Chapter 37 - Silent Night

IT IS CHRISTMAS EVE. I am the poster girl for cancer. I wear the classic, faded hospital gown. My face is obscured with a surgical mask, reading glasses, and my pink knit cap—pulled down over my ears and forehead. All I need is a red bow.

I'm still between chemo cycles, but dangerously low blood counts have landed me back in the hospital, my seventh stint as an inpatient in ten weeks. Transfusions begin immediately. A heart attack or brain hemorrhage could happen at any moment. *Fa la la la la....*

Light-headed, exhausted, and short of breath from even the smallest exertion—such as dressing or walking from one room to another—I lie immobile, again, in room 522. Lead moves through my veins. I can only mumble one or two-word answers to questions. Also wearing a surgical mask for my protection, Dan squeezes into my narrow hospital bed. We hold hands and watch *Christmas with the Kranks, National Lampoon Christmas,* and *Home Alone* while units of packed cells and platelets drip into me. At 2 AM, I convince my loving, loyal, and exhausted husband to go home. More blood and platelets are on the way. I feel deeply sorry for myself. And everybody else. I'm backsliding into *stinkin' thinkin'.*

It's early—maybe six—and still dark outside. I've slept a couple of hours. A nurse in a pointed red elf's cap comes in with another unit of packed cells.

"Can I go home when that one's empty?" I ask.

"Not yet."

"Maybe this afternoon?"

She shrugs.

Lying in the dim, silent room, I brood and fall into a new age hole. What if the message from the Center for Attitudinal Healing—*Health is inner peace. Healing is letting go of fear*—has even a smidgen of validity? What if my lousy attitudes and stockpiles of anxieties are the source of this misery? Allowing my mind to go the distance in a marathon of negativity, I obsess over how *I* might have caused this cancer. I'd made so many mistakes in my life; what if this lymphoma was the whopper of them all? Like an over-caffeinated stenographer, I record every one of my pitiful missteps:

*Why don't I have a real job: doctor, lawyer, or teacher?*

*Why didn't I save more money?*

*Why in my twenties did I sleep with guys I didn't love or even really care for?*

*Why didn't I give more time to Elspeth when she was little? Why did I send her away to play dates so I could do something I thought more interesting and valuable than spending hours with her, and Ken, and Barbie?*

Regret on top of regret, but the most insistent and clamoring: *Why wasn't I the wife Dan deserved, idealized, and hoped he had married?* Of course, he's never expressed this but after over twenty-five years of marriage I'm quite sure that his perfect wife brims with qualities I do not. Perpetually relaxed, Dan's perfect wife (DPW) doesn't fret about money or obsess about home decor. Willing to backpack and go to Harbin Hot Springs (clothing optional) where she will cheerfully cook in a communal kitchen and use a shared bathroom, DPW can live without down inserts in her pillows; she spends more time having sex with him and less time dragging him around to open houses; DPW wears her hair in the tousled style he loves, cooks him pork roasts, and doesn't harp about the benefits of a vegetarian diet.

*I could have done so much better. Why didn't I?*

The brooding sky mirrors the leaden color of the hospital walls and my mood. Discounting the nurse in the elf's cap, this could be any other sullen morning. I miss Dr. Arent. He would have worn a Santa suit today.

A wordless nurse hangs a new bag of platelets. I thank her. She nods and probably doesn't want to be here either.

Sitting up, I touch the cool, smooth bag. The gold platelets drip into the plastic tube connected to the IV in my hand. I trace the glassy droplets with my fingertip as they fall toward my body. *Do I even deserve all of this? Am I worth the effort, the trouble, the immense cost?*

My throat is tight with emotion, but I begin to hum and then sing, *"Silent night, holy night. All is calm, all is bright...."* The door opens and I stop singing. A smiling, heavyset African American woman, probably in her sixties, walks into the room. She delivers my breakfast tray, folds her hands, and sings, *"Round yon virgin...."*

I join her. *"...mother and child. Holy infant, so tender and mild. Sleeeep in heavenly peace. Sleeeep in heavenly peace."*

Her clear, deep voice thrills me. *"*

*Silent night, holy night! Shepherds quake at the sight. Glories stream from heaven afar. Heavenly hosts sing Alleluia! Christ, the Savior is born. Christ, the Savior is born."*

Smiling, with tears in my eyes, I say, "We're pretty good."

"Yes, that's right."

"Thank you for singing with me."

"It's the good Lord's birthday. Time to be joyful."

"Merry Christmas," I say.

"Merry Christmas to you."

She reaches into her pocket and hands me a candy cane.

"Thanks. My second gift," I say, pointing to the platelets.

## Chapter 38 - No Defense Against a Hurricane

NEW YEAR'S DAY. Like a personal time-share, I'm back in room 522 for another go-round of Hyper-CVAD. Exhausted and frail, my blood counts are again at the low, low levels. Outside the window, lethargic gray clouds float across the white winter sky.

"So, I understand that Natalia is recommending a stem cell transplant at Stanford," says Dr. Rivers, again on call for Dr. Greyz. He's a small man with a sharp nose and narrow eyes. He reminds me of a reptile. "It's a big procedure…." he says.

*Of course, it's a big procedure, so is Mantle Cell.*

"…and entails a rigorous preparation."

"She must think I can handle it," I say.

"Oh, I agree. You can."

I tense and feel that Dan and I are about to get information not shared with us by Dr. Greyz. And even though I don't *want* the transplant, I feel proprietary about my right to make that decision and grateful that Dr. Greyz is willing to do everything in her power to stop this lymphoma.

"What then?" I ask. "What are you saying?"

Rivers puts his hands in his lab coat pockets, then clears his throat.

"The outcomes are equivocal."

"The transplant doesn't come with a guarantee," says Dan. "We know that."

"How can I describe it? The transplant … it's really little more than a coat of paint that *might* help lengthen your remission." He almost sounds smug.

Dan glares at him. Suddenly chilled, I rub my arms with my hands. Paint chips and cracks with time. If the prep work isn't perfect, flaws show up quickly.

"Well, she seems to think you are a good candidate," he admits.

*What did that mean? That he didn't? That he thought I was too far gone for such heroics?*

"We trust her judgement," says Dan, his arms folded over his chest.

"Of course. Of course. I'm not trying to second-guess anyone."

"It's our best hope," says Dan. "Wouldn't you demand the same for your wife?"

"Yes, well, I'm sure things will work out." He seems to be backpedaling now, as if he realizes that he's stepped over a line.

*I'm sure things will work* out. *What does that even mean?*

I pull the white flannel blanket up around my neck and turn my head away from him.

"Let the nurses know if you need anything."

"What a jerk!" Dan exclaims. Rivers has barely left the room. "What a lame thing to say. I am so pissed."

A coat of paint is no defense against a hurricane.

# Chapter 39 - Relax

IN BETWEEN CYCLES FIVE and six of Hyper-CVAD, I make an appointment to see Dr. Gould. My last visit with him was the day of diagnosis and walking into his reception area now brings back the reined-in terror and surrealism of that September day. I'm here because of an itchy rash on my hands, arms, legs, and trunk that began with my last dexamethasone taper and has gotten worse. Wanting only to make a break for it, I sit and wait; my itchy hands clamp together.

When he enters the exam room, Dr. Gould smiles and hugs me. He's only ever touched me because it was his job, never with affection. He looks at me with compassion instead of neutrality. Maybe he is sorry that it was him. But maybe not. Perhaps he felt a tiny thrill at discovering something so unforeseen and, as it turned out, so potentially deadly. To make such a diagnosis is likely why he spent grueling years in medical school. This is what saving a life might look and feel like. (My Ob/Gyn had retired and never knew that in ignoring the lump I brought to his attention, he was missing an opportunity to save a life; but in his negligence, he almost took mine.)

"How are you?" Dr. Gould asks. "Putting up with the treatment?"

"Yeah. I'm okay. Except for this rash."

He squeezes my shoulder. While I don't ask, I assume that he's followed my progress by reading my computerized medical record. I would. Who wouldn't?

He looks at my hands and determines it's Dyshidrotic eczema. He prescribes high doses of antifungals and an antibiotic. The condition is likely brought on by stress. Really? He advises me to relax, and to avoid hot showers, hot tubs, or anything else that might dry out the skin. On that nightmarish day four months earlier, he'd also advised me to relax, but what else could he say?

This definition of Dyshidrotic eczema appears on the NIH website:

*Small fluid-filled blisters called vesicles appear on the fingers, hands, and feet. These blisters can be very itchy. They also cause scaly patches of skin that flake or get red, cracked, and painful.*

Sounds about right.

But after a week of treatment, the rash still itches like mad. I make an appointment with my dermatologist. Laurie and I see the same derm and have joked for years that she loves cutting and burning things off the skin. Sure enough, as soon as I sit down on the exam table, the doc grabs a scalpel. She makes a small incision in the skin on my left arm and using the side of the blade scrapes at one of my itchy blisters.

"Burrow," she mumbles.

She taps the scalpel blade onto a slide and peers at it under her microscope.

"Want to see what's going on?" she asks, sounding a bit puffed up.

Looking into the microscope, I jerk backwards, horrified to see an insect. Actually, it has eight-legs (a parasite) in contrast to six-legged insects. Not that the number of its disgusting little flailing legs matters one iota. This baby is ugly and resembles a cross between a turtle and a tank. Like a turtle, it has a bulbous body covered by a hard, tank-like shell. Unlike a turtle, dozens of sharp cones protrude from its back. Hair-like feelers emerge from its lower body, making it look capable of some very gruesome business. The diagnosis: Scabies.

Scabies infestation requires close physical contact with an infected person, but I've not had that. My dermatologist surmises that a scabies mite from Spirit or Harriet had probably landed on me. Usually, animal mites cannot take hold on humans—or produce only a mild itch that quickly disappears—but my severely immunocompromised condition gave the mighty mites a foothold. The little buggers took up residence under my skin, laid generations of eggs, and built themselves a thriving kingdom.

The infestation horrifies me. The hideous parasites strike me as an ingenious metaphor for the cancer that was born in my lymph nodes, thrived in my bone marrow, traveled throughout my blood stream, and colonized into malignant nodes all over my body in a nearly successful attempt to take over. But it also occurs to me how ultimately stupid the grisly cancer cell is: to wildly and unconsciously multiply and multiply until it kills the host that it is dependent on means the dim-witted cancer's own demise. Destruction for destruction's sake. Surely the mindless cancer cell must rank very low on the evolutionary scale. It exists only to kill and be killed. Sea cucumbers are Nobel Laureates by comparison.

I didn't think cancer would be like this. But who knows what cancer is supposed to be like?

# Chapter 40 - "The Hyper-CVAD Did the Tricks"

BY MID-JANUARY, I'VE COMPLETED six of the maximum eight rounds of Hyper-CVAD that any patient can tolerate. Results of a CT-PET scan show nearly full remission from Mantle Cell Lymphoma. The scan is mostly dark. Small gleaming nodes remain but the radiologist is not concerned. I can only wonder what the first scan looked like: Vegas? Times Square? Downtown Tokyo?

I sip the most expensive Chardonnay on the menu. I have an appointment with Dr. Greyz for a second bone marrow biopsy and I'm practicing preventive medicine. All about comfort food, I'm loving a bowl of home-made tomato soup and corn bread. In the chatter and buzz of this bright, busy café, I, in my Martha Stewart wig, look the same as the other women here. Ladies who are healthy, who lunch, who vacation.

"Do you remember when we swam out to Black Rock?" I ask Laurie.

"The most fun I've ever had being terrified."

"Me too." I take a long sip of cold wine.


*FIVE YEARS EARLIER, on a trip to Maui with our families, Laurie and I discussed whether we could swim out to Black Rock off Kaanapali Beach, and—more importantly—make it back. Neither of us was a great swimmer, but we were fit and young and adventurous.*

*The sea was calm that day. We talked each other out of our fear of the distance, the tides, the deep water. With fins, masks, and snorkels, we swam. And swam. As we neared Black Rock, the sun pierced deep into the clear, blue water, and the kaleidoscope of fish beneath us was breathtaking.*

*But better, much better, was the giant sea turtle that glided past. Letting the current take us, we followed the movement of his heavy flippers, the fine geometry of his shell. I was exuberant swimming with the graceful creature. Next to my newborn, he might have been the most beautiful thing I'd ever seen, well, except for Dan.*

*He surfaced, turned his head to look at us, and blinked.*

*I raised my face out of the water and looked shoreward. The beach umbrellas were smaller than the ones in our nightly Mai Tais. Laurie looked back too. How had we drifted so far? Were we caught in a rip tide? I took one last look at the beautiful sea creature.*

*We couldn't afford to panic. And didn't. Catching a wave shoreward whenever possible, we swam with deliberate strokes. Arm over arm, feet and legs kicking in the warm buoyant salt water, the sun hot on our backs. Eventually, we stumbled up onto the beach, our legs wobbly, but our spirits soaring. We couldn't stop smiling.*

*"I must be grinning like a clownfish, if a clownfish can grin," I said as I flopped down onto my towel.*

*Black Rock. A quarter mile out to sea from our hotel, fine linens, yoga on the beach, and sunset cocktails. We had ventured into a wilderness, been swept away, then returned.*

Cancer might be like swimming into deep water. It will give me a choice: to panic or to trust. I won't panic. I'll make steady progress and eventually get well and back to my beautiful, everyday life. But I won't be the same when I return because wild and indifferent cancer has swept me into its depths and currents and changed me into someone I can't even imagine yet.

Deep into our recollections of Maui, I forget about the biopsy until I glance at my watch. With a last swallow of Chardonnay, I down an Ativan. By the time Laurie and I walk into the office, I am cooperative—not exactly relaxed—but willing. I do not share my self-medicating with Dr. Greyz and ask if Laurie may come into the procedure room.

"Not one problem."

Although I clamp onto Laurie's hand with a death grip, this time is not as bad as the first. Dr. Greyz wrote in my medical record, *Pt tolerated procedure very well, no complic, min blood loss.* Yeah. Whatever helps.

THREE DAYS LATER, I wait alone in Dr. Greyz's warm, silent exam room. Outside the window, not even a cloud disturbs the blue winter sky. My body and mind are quiet. Maybe the fight has been knocked out of me, or perhaps I'm too tired to be scared. Smiling, Dr. Greyz sweeps into the room with my chart clasped to her chest.

"Oh, I am happy to see you. There is good news. Your bone marrow biopsy is negative for lymphoma."

We hug. She sets the folder down on her desk and gives it a little pat. "The Hyper-CVAD did the tricks."

"Yes," I smile and, while greatly relieved, also remember her first description of MCL as a cancer that responds well to treatment but has the nasty habit of coming right back. It's too soon to celebrate. I'm not in this struggle for a short-term gain and intend to reclaim the years that this cancer threatens to steal from me.

"It is time to send your brothers testing kits. I have a very good feeling on this."

"Me too," I say.

Dr. Greyz explains the two ways a bone marrow transplant can be achieved. One, called an autologous transplant, uses the patient's own irradiated stem cells to produce a new immune system. The second approach, an allogeneic transplant, uses donor cells that have never been cancerous to do the same. Before each transplant, the patient's previously cancerous immune system is obliterated with chemicals and radiation.

There are pros and cons with each approach. The autologous transplant is safer but less effective; the allogeneic is more effective against the cancer but carries the risk of graft versus host disease (GVHD). Even if one of my brothers is a perfect match, GVHD can occur. If that happens, their donated stem cells (the graft) perceive the host (me) as foreign and attempt to destroy it—sometimes successfully. But given that my bone marrow was nothing but cancerous paste at diagnosis, I get why Dr. Greyz insists on the allogeneic transplant and believes it is worth the GVHD risk.

"Leave your brothers' addresses with my receptionist. Stanford will send them testing kits."

I trust Dr. Greyz to act in my best interest. She has a youthful optimism that Dr. Rivers lacks. I have come so far and am ready to keep going. She and I are in this for a long-term win. We only need one of my brothers to get me to the finish line.


A WEEK LATER, IN THE cool afternoon January sun, I receive the bad news from Dr. Greyz. I walk home. Dan's car is in the driveway.

"Hey, where were you?"

"Walking." I hesitate, "Dr. Greyz called."

He doesn't take his eyes off me. We've both been waiting for her call.

"Neither Tom nor Randy is a match."

Dan sighs and lowers his head into his hands.

"And there's no one in the database."

"Jesus, I'm sorry."

"I don't believe it. I was sure Randy or Tom…." I begin to cry. Dan comes to me, gently removes my coat, and holds me.

"We still have Johnny," Dan says.

"I'll never find him," I say.

"We will."

"How?"

"I don't know. But we will."

The next day, I try the last phone number I have for Johnny. The one that the Doughnut Girls used to put us into contact. The number is disconnected, probably long gone. Knowing that it will be useless, I try Google and Facebook. Of course, he's not there.

Dan calls Randy who begins searching the many surf spots that Johnny frequented.

While Dr. Greyz never asks, "Why haven't you seen your brother in thirty years?" the question has many answers. Perhaps—like the fable of the elephant and the blind man—none of the reasons are completely true or accurate.

A few days later, Dr. Greyz phones and asks, "How about your third brother? You've come so far. We can't give up."

"All I know is that my brother cannot be found. There's nowhere else to look."

With every passing day, I fear that the cancer is doing its clever mathematical calisthenics of multiplying and dividing. Dr. Greyz is persistent and believes that I can find Johnny if I just keep trying. Dan and I avoid the discussion; we can't face talking about it.

# Chapter 41 - Holy Water from Lourdes

IF MY FRIEND, GAEL, could only carry two things, she would have a bottle of Chardonnay in one hand and a rosary in the other. She stands at my front door on a chilly and bright January afternoon, her platinum hair piled high on her head, a white wool coat on. She is a radiant vision in crimson lipstick offering me a platter of falafels, pita, and baba ganoush. She holds a cold bottle of Rombauer Chardonnay, her calling card. Party time. She walks in bringing a scent of lemon, cilantro, and perfume.

*Hello Darling. You look so beautiful.*

*You do too.*

*Can I help you carry something? I'm so glad you came.*

Gael is a hospice nurse and a believer in all that is spiritual and unseen. As girls, she and I bobby pinned our black-in-winter and white-in-summer mantillas onto our heads and walked together through our middle-class Los Angeles suburb of track homes, palm trees, and dichondra lawns to Saint Paul of the Cross to attend standing-room-only eleven o'clock Mass.

After years of dutiful—if not enthusiastic—church going, Gael and I reached our later teens and tossed the Mass and confession rituals. I had outgrown catechism and my mother—now more into sedatives and Vicodin than attending Mass herself—didn't seem to notice. Enter the Summer of Love, exit Saint Paul of the Cross Catholic Church. Then I had a fling into the wild Catholic girl thing, so popularized—and not hugely exaggerated—in the media. But thirty years later, Gael's return to faith was as swift and complete as her departure; and her life today is firmly guided by those still-vital Catholic roots. And Chardonnay.

We drink the expensive white wine and eat baba ganoush.

"Turns out I have to find my brother Johnny if I'm going to get out of this thing alive."

I'd never said that to anyone before. Not that bluntly about getting out alive.

"I mean, my doctor hasn't told me to get my affairs in order or anything like that, but she keeps telling me that I must find Johnny."

"Do you have any leads?"

"No. I've tried all of the contacts I had and Randy's scoured the Southern California beaches where Johnny surfed asking anyone who could have known him. We have nothing."

"I remember when I used to come over to your house, Johnny was so quiet. When I imagine him, it's as if he's standing against a wall trying to disappear."

"He had good reasons for wanting to disappear."

"How about a prayer to Saint Anthony?" asks Gael.

I laugh. "As a kid, I said lots of prayers to Saint Anthony to find lost books, barrettes, and Caesar, our un-neutered cat."

"How'd that go?"

"Not too bad, actually. Stuff usually turned up, including Caesar."

"I've lit a candle for you," she says, swirling the wine in her glass. "A tall votive with lovely religious images imprinted onto its sides. It's in my dining room and I will not let the flame go out until you are well."

"How tall is tall?"

"Fourteen or fifteen inches."

"I hope you don't have to buy too many."

We laugh again. "I've also asked the people in my parish to pray for you. There are hundreds of them."

"You know my belief system can't, let's say, hold a candle to yours; but what you are doing makes me feel protected, even safe. I don't know how to explain it."

"It's the Holy Spirit looking after you. That's what you are feeling."

"Or the Chardonnay."

We giggle again.

"Look how pretty," I say, moving my arm through a beam of light and tossing dust motes around. "I've got to play us something."

I rummage through a stack of CDs and play Elton John's *"Bennie and the Jets."* This is "our" song, the one Gael and I have danced to many times before. Back in the living room, Gael is already on her feet. We give it all we've got, rocking out through the sunlight, the dust motes, and Elton John's irresistible words and melody.

After the song is over, we hug like two people who've been searching for each other for a long time. I pant from the glorious effort.

"A friend of mine brought this from Lourdes. I want you to have it," Gael says pulling a small glass bottle from her purse.

Although I've never seen a bottle of the liquid itself, the healing powers of holy water from Lourdes got frequent mention in our Catholic girlhoods. The clear glass container is visually unassuming but oddly provocative.

"Will you give me a blessing?"

Standing face to face in front of the French doors, sunlight pouring in on us, I close my eyes. Gael rests her hands on my warm shoulders, and I sense the pure and deep intension of her prayers. How can I explain or describe this? Is it grace? Healing? Like the pink mist, her prayers leave me calm and stronger.

"You will need to be brave, but I believe you will be well again."

I open my eyes. Gael smiles and presses a cool drop of holy water onto the tiny scar on my neck where the cancerous node had been removed. I shiver and feel cleaner, as if I'd just had a quick douse in a cold river.

"I'll pray for you to find Johnny."

"Yeah, baby," I reply.

As a person who chucked her religious upbringing and didn't look back, I am amazed at being so moved by a prayer and a drop of water.

Between the wine, the dancing, and the water from Lourdes, I feel I've been delivered. I don't know where, but somewhere new and brighter.

# Chapter 42 - Zaba What?

MY FRIEND ANNE IS BREATHLESS, "I've heard about this thing. It might help find your brother," she says.

I grip the phone listening to her words rush over each other.

"A woman I know is freaking out about this search engine that finds people and publishes their names, ages, addresses, and phone numbers online unless they opt out."

"What is it?"

"It's called ZabaSearch. It's pretty invasive. They don't tell you that you *need* to opt out. I'm going to search it for Johnny."

We hang up. I feel no spark of hope, just confusion. It's been six weeks since finishing chemo and my last CT-PET scan. Pressing the sides of my neck and under my arms, I cannot detect any lumps but worry that the cancer cells might be creating vast colonies inside my bone marrow.

There is another check for a donor in the international database. Still no one, and the odds are slim to none that someone will appear. But I work a little, cook, feel better. Not like before the lymphoma, but so much stronger than in the hospital. Once in a while I forget about the whole damn thing.

Late afternoon the next day the doorbell rings. I lean backwards the smallest bit when I see Anne holding neatly typed papers that rustle in the breeze. Taking the crisp pages, I flip through them. The sight of my brother's name over and over feels like a weight sinking from my heart to my stomach. I roll the pages into a tight tube. If my brother's phone number is in these pages, I've just crossed a threshold, a point of no return. I'm afraid. I cannot afford fear.

"Thank you for doing this. It's very kind of you."

"Tell me what happens," says Anne.

Drumming the rolled pages against my thigh, I pace. Dan will be home soon. I walk into my office and put the pages face down in a wicker basket under a stack of folders. I don't mention them to Dan.

Two days go by until I dig out the list and step outside my office doors into the backyard and a steely blue day. A chilly February breeze flutters the leaves of the Fan Palm and the papers in my hand. Of course, I've been thinking about the list; I just couldn't face it yet. The morning feels charged with too much nitrogen or oxygen. So many names and phone numbers. I'm unsettled, agitated. I want something big from someone I don't know anymore, someone who might be dead, or....

Breathing deeply, I try to calm down. Dr. Greyz has warned me about getting nervous.

There are over forty names on the list with addresses and phone numbers. All but one of the contacts are in Southern California, which both frightens and encourages me as that's where Johnny's always lived. The third page contains only one entry with no address but from the phone number it cannot be him. The area code is for the next county just miles north of here. Johnny was always a beach boy.

Sipping water to moisten my throat, I glide a ChapStick over my dry lips but fear that I am a faker, worse, a user. No preparation can make me deserving.

If I'm going to make these calls, I must get beyond my decades-old guilt of not helping Johnny. Today, I'm looking for him and will ask some huge thing that I don't begin to understand. Why do I think I deserve his help? Could I have done more for him? I'm back to the same old question without an answer.

I look at a family portrait of the three of us. I owe Dan and Elspeth. The least I can do is call the names that Anne was kind enough to find. If I don't, I'll fail everyone, including Dr. Greyz. What's the worst that can happen?

I straighten my shoulders and decide what I'm going to say.

"Hi, my name is Susan. Susie. Do you have a sister with that name?"

With trembling fingers, I dial the first number, and the second, and then all forty from the first two pages. People answer. Some are kind; some are brusque. No one has a sister named Susan. Machines answer. I leave messages that are not returned or if they are, it's not my Johnny. I put the list back in the basket and at dinner tell Dan. Another disappointment. Another dead end.

The next day, I have an appointment at Stanford but before Dan and I leave, I call the last number on the third page of the list. I let it ring and ring. No answer. No machine.

Twenty-one tubes of blood, my personal best, are taken from my VAP at the Stanford clinic this morning. Why do I keep coming back? I have no donor. All of this seems pointless and a waste of time. Yet I am signed up to be part of a clinical trial and wonder, *Am I the defendant or the plaintiff? Who is the judge, the jury? Am I guilty or innocent?*

When we get home, I'm exhausted and climb into bed. But my compulsion for thoroughness gets the better of me. The sun is down. I turn on my bedside lamp and pick up Anne's list, certain that my effort will be useless. Harriet discovers the perfect location against my thigh and begins kneading and purring. Downstairs, Dan clangs around in the kitchen. Winter hangs on in the cold, February sky but spring is in the wings, ready.

I dial the last number again. It rings and rings. No answer. I hang up, then wait and think, *Just one more time.* I redial and my cell phone buzzes in my hand.

## Chapter 43 – In Johnny's Own Words
## Willits, 2006

I PUSH OPEN THE GATE, creaking with age; a burlap sack of foraged, edible mushrooms is slung over my shoulder. I sigh. The phone's ringing. I'm not expecting to hear from anyone and hope that the threatening crank calls aren't starting up again. I decide to ignore it but then, still carrying the sack, I remove my muddy boots and open the backdoor dropping the bag inside. By the time I reach the phone, the caller has hung up. I go back outside, relieved to be rid of any interruption to my well-deserved dinner and evening.

I put my fingers to my face and breathe in the sweet earthy smell of the mushrooms, a scent that will likely remain on my hands for another day. I push my shoulders back and sigh again. I'd walked miles today and am feeling the warm seduction of fatigue. Across the expansive yard, my chickens, Buffy and Pepper, barrel toward me like chubby roadrunners, flapping their wings, excited to see me.

The hens crowd around my feet and I feel satisfied after my long day. I look around my backyard and think that I'm lucky to be living here in Willits.

I pick up Buffy, her feathers as soft and yellow-white as the caps of the Chanterelles I'd harvested.

"This place suits us, doesn't it girl?"

Buffy nestles into my body while Pepper dances around trying to get my attention.

There, just next to the wire deer fence bordering my backyard is Billy Bob O'Binkley, reclining on his donated mattress with a soiled canvas tarp suspended above it, his camping spot for the past five years.

"What's for dinner tonight, old boy?" asks the elderly Billy Bob.

"Pasta with Shaggy Manes."

"Nice to have a little something before our repast. My Olde English is getting low."

"All the hot meals I feed you aren't enough?"

"Not that I don't appreciate them, old boy, you know I do, but man does not live by bread alone."

I reach into my pocket for a ten-dollar bill and hand it through the wire fence to Billy Bob who grunts, "Thanks, man," but doesn't get up.

The phone rings again. I frown and put Buffy back on the ground. Inside, I tuck my hair behind my ear and pick up the receiver.

"Johnny?" It's a woman's voice I don't recognize and feel a moment of relief that it's probably not a prankster. They're always guys.

"Yes?" I run my hand down my graying goatee.

"Do you have a sister named Susan?"

"Yeah?"

"It's me, Susie."

The perfection of the day drains away. I haven't spoken to my sister in decades. How did she track me down? What does she want?

"I'm sorry. It's been so long. That's my fault," she says.

"Hey, there's no fault."

"How are you?"

"I'm fine."

"I thought you would still be in Southern California," she says.

"Nor Cal boy now."

The question hangs heavily between us.

"I'm sure you're wondering why I called."

"Yeah. I guess so."

"I'm sick."

"No." I feel afraid of what she's going to say.

"Lymphoma."

"I'm … sorry."

"I need a bone marrow transplant. Randy isn't a match, neither is Tom, and there's no one in the international database."

Outside my kitchen window, the ash and apple trees—in shadow against the silver sky—show a few early budding leaf clusters peeking out from moss-covered branches. Buffy and Pepper are eating something out of Billy Bob's hand which annoys me. He knows I am careful about their diets.

"There's no one else to ask."

"What do you need?"

"I need you to be tested. To see if we're a match."

"I'll do whatever I can."

"You will?"

"Of course," I say with more confidence than I feel. My voice wavers.

"Thank you, Johnny. Stanford will send you a kit. You just need to take it to a local lab where they will get a blood sample and mail it back. Thank you. Thank you so much," Susie says.

I give her my address but as I hang up, I feel as if I've just been clocked. I wander back outside and pick up Pepper.


THREE DAYS LATER I RECEIVE A LETTER.


*February 19, 2006*

*Dearest Johnny,*

*Thanks so much for talking with me. My phone call must have been startling after so long. And an even bigger shock to be needed for such a possibly profound job.*

*By the time you get this, you will likely have received the testing kit from Stanford. I deeply appreciate your help. I fear that without a transplant, my* chances of survival are pretty slim. Even with the transplant, I might only have a few years.

I don't mean to be pessimistic or morbid, but I'm afraid it is simply the case. My "assignment" is to make the very most of each day (not unlike anyone else's, of course) but for me, those days might be fewer than I'd thought or hoped.

I've enclosed some recent photos of my family.

There is so much more to say, but please forgive me if I keep this brief. I cannot write any more today.

Love you always,

Susan

# Chapter 44 - "Everything Happens for a Reason"

THE DAY AFTER THE LETTER ARRIVES, Susie calls me back. We're a perfect match. I'm confused. I want to help my sister, but there are a lot of issues that could make seeing each other awkward, at best.

I enter my indoor marijuana garden, in the second bedroom of my home, and take a deep breath. The plants—halfway into their flowering stage—give off the sharp, sweet odor of terpenes, like some exotic perfume. I never get tired of that scent. The four 1000-watt halide light bulbs hum as the fans swivel back and forth gently blowing filtered air onto the plants. I touch the newly forming flowers, sticky with a diamond-like coating of dense, fragrant resins. This potent Indica/Sativa hybrid, known as "Blueberry Bubblegum," will bring $3,000 a pound when mature—assuming they have the correct nutrients, light, ventilation, and water. If all goes well, I'll end up with about three pounds of product ready to be snapped up by eager clients. But growing high-quality ganja is not a chore for beginners. If I'm helping my sister, almost two hundred miles away in Stanford, what will happen to these plants and the income I must have from them?

In the living room I look at the 100-gallon terrarium that houses my tropical New Caledonian Giant Geckos. They also need specialized care. Billy Bob is not up to any of this.

I'm so damned confused. *Torn*. I walk back outside and my hens glance off of each other as they scramble toward me. I lodge Pepper under an arm and pace around the backyard. The new soil for replanting my garden has just been delivered. The pile of fine black earth will have to wait. I'll need to be in the Bay Area for a week, maybe more. I look around and know I am tied to this house, my plants, and animals; but it is a leash that I love.

It's getting late and I feel the desire. I want my high-quality cannabis and the two glasses of wine I enjoy, daily, at happy hour. I pour a glass of red wine and drink deeply. I sit on my back step with Buffy and Pepper on each side of me. The wine is good. It relaxes me.

"Hey, old boy," says Billy Bob, "you look a little down in the mouth."

"Yeah. I'm going away for a while and I'm worried about things around here."

"No worries, my friend. I'll take care of it."

"Nice of you to offer," I say but wonder, *What good will a semi-conscious security guard be? He can't even feed himself.*

"Have to give this up too," I say, holding my wine glass up for Billy Bob to see.

"Oh man, that's tough." He takes a hefty swig out of his 40-ounce bottle of Olde English Malt Liquor.

"I'm not gonna cheat and get high, but I do like my nightly wine and weed."

"I hear you, brother."

In the kitchen, I sit at the table, pour another glass, and call my landlords, Jeff, and Kathy. Kathy answers and when I'm done with my story, she immediately offers to take care of my indoor pot garden and all the animals.

"That's very generous of you."

"Oh, Johnny, we have all kinds of help. I'll get my nephews to take care of your hens and geckos, and my mom will tend the plants."

"You think your mom is up to the task, with the pot?"

"My mom's 80, and she's no newbie. Every year, for Christmas money, she grows good-quality cannabis in her backyard just north of town. Her green thumb has never failed her."

"Well, that sounds great."

I'm still feeling very unsettled about the whole situation, but things do seem to be falling into place.

"And Jeff and I will drive you to San Rafael."

"Oh no. I'm fine getting there on my own."

"I won't hear of it. We'll take you."

They are captivated by the story of the youngest black sheep brother (me) reuniting with my long-estranged sister to hopefully help cure her of a lethal cancer. They treat me as both a hero (which makes me self-conscious and very uncomfortable) and paradoxically like a child incapable of making even the smallest decision for myself. While I don't drive and would have preferred to make this journey on a Greyhound bus, giving me time to think and get used to the idea of seeing Susie, I deeply need and appreciate their help with my plants and animals.

Two days later, as we travel through the green winter landscape of Northern California, I brood over how I will find my sister and try to remember how old we were when we last saw each other. Late teens for me. Susie was in her mid-twenties. Thirty years ago.

From the front seat, Kathy announces, "Everything happens for a reason!"

As I'm sitting in the back, she can't see me rolling my eyes. I've heard her spout this line of reasoning before and think, *Here we go again.*

"You mean that my sister's illness and our match is fate and all predetermined?"

"Absolutely. There are powers far greater than ourselves."

"Yes. People get cancer, need help, and contact someone they haven't spoken to in a long time. Throw in a coincidence or two—and as a rationalist—that's enough for me!"

"Oh, Sweetie, you just don't see the big picture."

Kathy thinks I am just too dim to follow her logic; well, it's not really logic is it?

"What I see is you and Jeff being incredibly generous, and I appreciate it very much."

"Oh, Sweetie," Kathy says again and shakes her head.

As we get closer to Marin County, I become more nervous. My jaw is tight and as much as I am determined to help my sister, I'd like for all of this to just be over. I shift around in my seat. I don't want to create any problems for her or her husband. I don't have money or culture. I'm beat up around the edges. What will she think of me? We are probably very different. But what the hell? I can only be who I am and smile as I remember the Oscar Wilde quote: "Be yourself, everybody else is taken."

I hope she'll offer me a glass of wine when we get there.

# Chapter 45 - Susan and Johnny, Reunited, 2006

A WEEK AGO, I'D SAT ON my bed, staring out the window into the cold, dark sky. Harriet's tiny purring body was warm against my leg. Twice I'd dialed the last number on the list Anne had given me and gotten no answer. Ready to toss the papers aside, I thought, just one more time, and redialed. I let it ring and ring before he answered. I knew immediately. Soft, melodic, and almost breathy, Johnny's simple hello was childlike and wise at the same time. A kind person without sharp edges, someone who despite the cruel knocks that life has dealt him, has no hardness or bitterness. When he answered the phone, the past became present, as if years had gone by and no time at all.

And then, for him to be a perfect match.

How karmic, how poetic, that it is Johnny, the brother I tried to protect and defend. How complicated it all is. I'd found a brother who didn't want to be found. Being in touch with him reminds me—and, I'm certain, him—of the old days, days that I, and I'm sure Johnny, have tried to forget. And now I'm asking him to do something that neither of us understands. Beyond the transplant, I'm asking him to see me again, to come back into my life.

Another small cut—after I told Tom, Randy, and our mother that I'd found Johnny, no one asked for his address or phone number. Nor did he ask for theirs.


I'VE FINISHED MAKING DINNER. The table is set. The house is clean and quiet. Too quiet. The wait for Johnny is making me edgy. I go upstairs. The woman in the dark blond, layered-cut, Martha Stewart wig who stares back from the bathroom mirror is only a replica of myself, an artificially garnished copy without eyebrows or eyelashes. Screw it. Off comes the damned wig. Johnny will arrive soon and be reunited with the current me—the woman who is unadorned, needy, and bald. *What will he think of me? I of him? Who is he? Who am I?*

I fuss over what to wear. I don't want to appear too formal or too sloppy. It is just a dinner at home. It is just a reunion with a brother I haven't seen in three decades. I want to make the right impression, strike the proper tone. I decide on good jeans, a white sweater, and low-heeled gray suede boots. No jewelry other than my wedding ring and the diamond stud earrings I always wear. Nothing more.

I flinch at the ring of my cell phone. Dan's name lights the screen.

"Hey, Honey. Is Johnny there?"

"Where are you? Why aren't you home?"

"What's wrong?"

"What if he chain smokes? Or swears all the time? What if we can't talk to each other? How weird would that be?"

"I'll be home soon."

"When?"

"Soon."

Downstairs, I pace the living room.

*What if he scares me? What if he doesn't like who I am? Thinks I sold out, lost my soul in a vicious scramble for money.*

I pour a glass of wine and swallow half an Ativan that I snared from the hospital. I turn and look out the French doors. The treetops quiver. I step outside and fold my arms around myself. Metallic-colored clouds streak across the wintery sky. I breathe in the cold air and feel it enter and settle my body. And there, the first fuzzy evening star. I love the winter light, so clean and piercing.

Just after 5 PM there is the tentative knock. Coming back inside, I run a palm over my warm head. Spirit disappears down the hallway into Elspeth's bedroom. With a shaky hand, I grasp the front door latch. The sky gleams silver behind Johnny's head. I smile and look at his kindly face seeing my little brother, now a middle-aged man.

"Johnny."

He smiles and pulls his long, wavy, salt-and-pepper hair behind his back and puts his arms around me. Feeling weak with gratitude and relief, I shudder then weep into his chest.

He pats my back. "It's okay, Sis. It's okay."

I look at his face again. "I can't believe you're here."

I wipe tears from my cheeks. Behind Johnny, a man coughs. A woman gives a little wave.

"Hi," I say. "I'm Johnny's sister, Susan—Susie."

"This is Kathy and Jeff," Johnny says. "They're my friends and drove me down from Willits."

They're about fifty and unremarkably dressed. I figure them for mild-mannered Republicans who are involved in church charities and work with their local Chamber of Commerce. In his tie-dyed tee-shirt and long hair, Johnny looks like Jeff and Kathy's wayward hippy adoptee. I am momentarily alarmed thinking that he needs a driver and what that might mean.

"Come in. Please."

"No thanks," says Kathy. "This is the time for you and Johnny to get reacquainted. We have dinner and hotel reservations in San Fran."

I am not relieved to see Johnny's friends go and am concerned that my brother and I might not have anything to say to each other. He comes inside, carrying nothing.

"Do you have a bag?"

"No, got my toothbrush in my pocket. That's all I need."

I wonder about a change of clothes but say nothing.

"Can I get you a drink? A glass of wine?"

"Red's good."

"Please," I say gesturing toward the living room.

In the kitchen, I text Dan, "Home soon?"

I pour Johnny a glass of wine, pick up mine, and sit across the coffee table from him. Although it's February and cold, he wears no jacket, just a tee shirt with a hole in the sleeve. He's missing a front tooth. A tooth he had the last time I'd seen him. The lamp light gives the room a warm glow.

"Nice place."

I take a long sip of wine. "I don't know where to start."

"How about today?"

Grateful that he's not dredging up the past, my shoulders relax.

"Yes. Okay. I—Dan and I—have a daughter. I sent you her picture."

"Cool to be an uncle. Tell me about her."

Ten minutes later, Dan walks in. Dressed in the navy-blue Armani suit I'd bought him for Christmas and carrying a leather briefcase, he looks as though he resides in a different universe from the one that contains my brother. But the moment is affectionate, like a homecoming. Johnny stands, pulls his hair behind his shoulders, and holds out his hand. Dan steps forward and embraces him, while his briefcase presses against Johnny's back.

Covering my face, I whisper, "Please, please," and "thank you, thank you," behind my hands.

"What you're doing, Johnny," Dan starts, then clears his throat. "It means … you mean … so much to us."

"I hope I can help. There's more testing."

"You sure look healthy," I say, although I know that he has been—maybe still is—into drugs. Heart disease and addiction run in our family … and, apparently cancer.

## Chapter 46 - The Snake Charmer

FOR DINNER, I SERVE A homemade marinara over linguini and clams and Dan says, "Tell me about Willits."

"Well, it's a couple hours north of here. Once it was a busy logging center, now it's on the skids with a marijuana economy that barely supports the locals."

"What do you do up in the redwoods?" Dan asks.

"Odd jobs for Jeff and Kathy. On a farm. You know, marijuana. And I have my own plants and sell high-quality cannabis, some to a medical marijuana club in L.A., but mostly to older folks with chronic pain who prefer pot to the opioids."

While not surprised, I tense at his mention of marijuana. Why does my brother have to be involved in an illicit product, an illegal pastime? I cannot fathom the two middle-aged, plain-vanilla-looking Jeff and Kathy as drug lords, well, pot growers. I'd smoked some pot in my twenties but never liked the effects. I either got paranoid, sleepy, or ate everything I could find. It never made sense to me.

"I also raise rare geckos and send them around the country."

"Wow. Who wants them?" I ask.

"Collectors and people trying to save them from extinction."

"What a wonderful thing to do, saving geckos. Saving me is pretty freaking huge too." I smile at my brother. "He's always been an animal lover."

"Tell me about it," says Dan.

"When I was eleven and twelve, I used paper route money to purchase my first Southeast Asian Tokay Gecko. He had blue and orange spots and was about 10 inches in length with large gold eyes. To appear as large as possible, he would raise up high on his four legs,"—Johnny lifts up in his seat and elevates his shoulders—"then swell his body with air, open his large mouth and lunge at any perceived threat, all the while emitting a loud sound resembling a cross between a dog's bark and the quack of a duck. The fact that he could walk across a vertical pane of glass or upside down across a ceiling was a buyer's point for me. I also talked Mom into getting me an iguana for Christmas as she wasn't as frightened of lizards as she was snakes—of which she had a full-on phobia."

I shake my head. "Wow, you've got your gecko details down."

"So, where did you keep them?" asks Dan.

"In the garage on an old kitchen table, housed in large aquariums. To keep them warm, I used aquarium heaters in quart jars of sand. I bought crickets and meal worms for the Tokay, and the iguana ate greens. He loved dandelions, fruits, and veggies. Mom, of course, didn't care for the reptiles and kept her distance. To her credit, however, she allowed me to house a couple of others in cages."

"I'm surprised that she went along with any of this," I say.

"Well,"—Johnny looks down at his plate—"she assumed I only had lizards. In fact, there were a number of snakes swelling my collection. I never mentioned them to her."

"Uh-oh." I shake my head and think this is exactly the sort of thing that Beverly would put into the "You Just Can't Trust Him Bucket," and apparently there is some evidence for that.

I've had enough but pour more wine for all of us. No one objects.

"I had a friend named Sammy, and one of our favorite things was to wander around the La Mirada Swap Meet on weekend mornings."

"I was there once or twice. It was pretty rough," I say.

"Yeah, it was. Sammy and I would sneak in through a hole in a chain link fence and spend hours cruising around looking at all the crazy stuff and the eccentric folks. You could buy fireworks and even Mexican pot or peyote. It was the late 60s and vendors were playing and selling 8-track tapes from groups like Hendrix, The Doors, Crosby, Stills and Nash, and early works of Carlos Santana. All very heady stuff for us preteens."

"I met Jim Morrison once, at a party at UCLA. We only got introduced, but it was such a buzz," I say, remembering Morrison's deep-set eyes staring at me in a dark, crowded hallway, him mumbling *Hi*.

"One of the vendors had a kiosk that was a veritable candy shop of colubrids."

Colubrid. It must be a snake but I've never heard the word.

"I ended up buying a lot from him. Every penny from my paper route went into my snake collection."

My shoulders twitch involuntarily at the thought of all those scaly creatures. Head tilted, Dan stares at Johnny, mesmerized.

"So, you were loading up on snakes in the garage and Mom had no idea?" I ask.

"Right. I was surprised, but she didn't seem to notice the growing number of cages."

"I get why she wouldn't have liked her garage full of snakes," I say.

"I ended up with a reticulated python more than nine feet long."

"What? How did you hide a nine-foot python?" I ask, feeling a little queasy. I shoot a look of "yuck" toward Dan.

"Also, an African ball python—both were rare in collections then—a red-tailed boa, a corn snake, a large and boisterous yellow rat snake, a vicious Cooks tree boa, a blue racer." Johnny looks toward the ceiling, as if trying to remember.

"A melanistic/black hognose snake, a huge gopher snake that tried to strangle me after I placed it around my neck, a long-nosed snake, a desert glossy snake, two species of leaf-nosed snakes, a rear-fanged desert night snake, a pair of granite night lizards, a pair of banded geckos, three noisy Tokay geckos, a tarantula, two scorpions, and a few others."

"What? How can you possibly recall all of those?" I ask.

"The names of the rest of my collection escape me."

"And how could you have hidden them?"

Johnny smiles and shrugs.

I am creeped out by the image of all those reptiles writhing around in the garage and am equally impressed that the names of all those varieties just roll off Johnny's tongue.

"When the cages began to fill up the back of the garage, Mom started to pay attention; also, the growing electricity bills were noticed. But it was the California Lyre snake, *Trimorphodon Biscutatus,* semi-poisonous with opisthoglyphic fangs, that was the end of most of my collection. The Lyre snake—a rare and secretive nocturnal denizen of caves and areas of huge boulders—feeds on bats and lizards and paralyzes its prey by injecting it with a venom from fangs in the rear of its mouth."

*Trimorphodon Biscutatus, opisthoglyphic, denizen. Where did this vocabulary come from? Johnny had always been super smart, but he sounds like a biology text.*

I'm nervous and wonder if he is too. Maybe that's why all the scientific terminology.

"My Lyre snake was about two feet long. Somehow, it escaped its cage and instead of heading off to any number of places outside the garage, it chose to enter the house. How it got in, I don't know. Its next unfortunate move was to crawl into Mom's bedroom, up the side and onto the bed, then directly over her midsection while she was watching M.A.S.H. and eating cookies and ice cream."

"No," I say. Dan and I are now laughing.

"Mom screamed. I ran into her bedroom. She was hysterical, 'A snake just crawled over me. Find it and get rid of it and get rid of all those horrible creatures in the garage.' I looked around and found my prized snake in the bathroom, coiled up near the toilet, and took it back into its cage in the garage. She was still yelling.

"After that, I gave away most of my collection, but smuggled the two pythons, at about nine feet each, and Sylvia, the boa, around the same size, into my dresser drawers where they rested most happily on pilfered heating pads. I misjudged that Mom would find them. Of course, she eventually did. I continued to move the snakes to different areas but am a bit unclear, all these years later, as to where they ultimately ended up. I placed this unfortunate incident into my mental file of 'Why Does This Bad Stuff Always Happen to Me?'"

Dan is laughing with his hand over his mouth, while I glimpse something about my brother that makes me uncomfortable: he kept getting more and more snakes, *knowing* how much our mother feared them. Collecting so many snakes would be another huge reason for her dislike of Johnny, but he did it anyway. Looked at another way, maybe the snakes were a sign of his emotional equilibrium, an expression of autonomy, the not unwarranted F-you comeback.

"Did you really think that Mom wouldn't notice three, nine-foot snakes in your dresser?"

Johnny shrugs.

"That's one hell of a story," says Dan smiling. "Poor Beverly."

I bet there is much more I don't know about Johnny. When he was eleven and starting to collect all these snakes, I'd just graduated high school and was out on my own. I'd never known about the reptiles.

"But why so many snakes?" I ask.

"I got lost in them. They were a ready escape from the vicissitudes inside the house."

*Vicissitudes,* I think. What an odd word to choose. I wonder if Johnny is trying to impress me, trying to shield me from other words that might have been more descriptive: *contempt, disgust, punishment.* While his story makes me laugh, I am also on the verge of tears. I've wanted so much more for him than reptiles and marijuana. Could I have done more? I can't let go of the question. At some deep recess, I knew this is what his life would look like. And that I wouldn't like it, yet I'd done little to help or change it. If I ever could.

# Chapter 47 - You Can't Judge Him

IN THE CAR THE NEXT MORNING, on our way to Stanford, I ask Johnny about his missing tooth.

"It was a bike accident. Couple of years back."

"Ouch."

"Wasn't bad."

"We'll see if we can get that fixed," I say.

"No worries."

I want to help him, but is a new tooth for him or for me?

We arrive at the Cancer Center where he goes off for a day of what I imagine will be rigorous testing. Dan and I wait for my appointment with a radiation oncologist.

"Your brother's a great guy," Dan says. "but a little forgetful. He didn't bring any underwear, so I gave him a pair of my boxers."

"I'm not surprised. He had no overnight bag, and this morning he asked me if I thought he should take a shower."

"Really?"

"Yeah. I told him that a shower would be a good idea."

"He's his own man."

"What else did you think of him?" I ask.

"He's kind. And terrifically smart."

"He says he reads the *L.A. Times* from front to back every day."

"Funny, huh?" says Dan. "To be isolated and so in touch."

"Yeah. But his life depresses me. He's spent so much time in the drug world."

"You can't judge him for that."

"Why can't I?"

"It's his life."

"And one I don't want for my little brother. I don't care what other people do, but he's my family. What if he goes to jail?"

"He won't go to jail."

"How can you know that?"

"I can't. But you have to face the fact that his business is drugs."

"I don't *have* to face anything. He's my brother. I can feel any way I want."

"Suit yourself."

"Damn right I will."

I'm furious. Easy for Dan to be uninvolved. He and Johnny have no history, no connection except for this transplant. And Dan has a more easygoing attitude toward drugs than I do. In my mind, using is one thing, selling is quite another.

Then I wonder if I'm the one with the problem. Will my judgement stand in the way of us ever being close? Probably, but I won't be able to help it, no matter how much I wish I could.

We are called into our appointment and I cool down.


THE UPSHOT OF THE ALL-DAY Stanford testing: Johnny is healthy enough to withstand the donor protocol. Whatever it is. I am as grateful as I am afraid. For both him and me.

On the drive home, I ask Johnny about his relationship with Tom.

"Well, there's not a lot to say. We lived in different universes. At four years older than I, we had no shared interests, and never had one 'real' conversation between us. He did hurl a few low-level sarcastic comments at me, but maybe I deserved them as I was certainly no prize either. Just a pesky little brother who invaded his room, played his records, read his underground comix—pretty intense stuff for a preteen—and thumbed through his *Playboy* magazines. Hey, I was just reading the articles. I also 'borrowed' his ten-speed bike without asking, which did earn his enmity."

The car is warm and stuffy. From the back seat, I ask Dan to turn on some air.

"Tom had his band, and they rehearsed in our garage super loud."

"I remember the band," I say.

"So, I felt I had to remove all of my reptiles when he practiced, which resulted in scorn from him. He said, 'Snakes don't have ears! They can't hear!' True, but they are very sensitive to vibrations and I didn't want to stress them out, which he thought was really stupid."

I can picture Johnny, patiently moving the cages into a little-used side yard, trying to protect his buddies, while still hiding them from Mom.

"Tom liked to grow houseplants, and one day I noticed he had a nice Coleus in his room. I was about fourteen and had read that the Mazatec tribes of Southern Mexico chewed Coleus to create visions. That sounded like tremendous fun. I basically denuded the plant. The taste was terrible and I received no visionary reward whatsoever, only mild stomach cramps, and disdain from Tom as he fingered me as a most likely suspect."

"Poor Tom." Dan and I are laughing. "Of course, he knew you did it. Do you know anything about him now?" I ask.

"No."

"At nineteen, Tom was in love something fierce, and his girlfriend wanted to get married. He said they were too young. So, very quickly, she married someone else and had a daughter. Tom stayed a bachelor, and by the time he was in his early thirties, had become a chemist and pretty reclusive. Maybe he never got over his girlfriend leaving," I say, "or Dad walking out."

Johnny's silent, as if he doesn't want to touch this topic, but I move it forward. "Once, I tried to talk to him about our childhood. He said, 'It's past. Over and done.' Even though he dismissed it, I don't believe that he was unscathed."

"Hmm," Johnny says, and I drop the conversation.


ON SATURDAY, FRIENDS PUT on a party for me, a bon voyage. I don't know who organized it. Dozens of people bring piles of food. Music plays. There are flowers. I am fragile, bald, and immensely happy.

Early in the evening, a woman in a large, floppy hat and huge sunglasses knocks on the door. I open it and Elspeth flies into my arms. I had no idea my daughter was coming and am more verklempt than ever. Elspeth has never met her Uncle Johnny and they become an immediate mutual admiration society: likely the most beautiful girl in the room with the guy who might feel a little out of his depth in this sophisticated crowd. But he mingles, often with his hand partially over his mouth obscuring the missing tooth. I drink a lot of wine. Johnny tells me later that he has never seen so many stunning women in one place.

The next morning Kathy and Jeff arrive to take him back to Willits.

"I'll see you in two weeks," I say.

"I'll be back."

We hug and I whisper, "Thank you," into his neck.

Johnny will be back. He will not abandon me as our father had. He and I are held together with stronger glue than that. Not making the same ruinous mistakes that our parents did is our own beautiful rebellion.

# Chapter 48 - Remove All Teeth Affected by Gum Disease

A BOX FROM STANFORD ARRIVES; its size and weight suggest it contains a phone directory from the Greater New York Metro Area. Inside is the *Allogeneic Blood and Marrow Transplant Guidebook* from Stanford. I wrestle it out of the box and scan the table of contents. I love checklists and go right to that page. Seems they've thought of everything from identifying a caregiver to changing the air filter on the home furnace. Practice drinking three quarts of water every day. Have a dental exam. All cavities should be filled and any teeth affected by gum disease should be removed. *Removed?* Plan for pet care. Obtain a medical alert bracelet. Review and update your Advanced Directive. Check, check, and check. Oh, the air filter, I don't know. Otherwise, good.

After reading the checklist, I scan the table of contents again and see Sexual Activity for Women:

*Both men and women report low interest in sexual activity. In most cases interest or sexual desire returns about six months after transplant. You may resume sexual activity once your platelet count is above fifty thousand.*

As my count is currently four thousand, I have a ways to go.

*Ovaries stop producing hormones ... Vaginal dryness may occur because of chemotherapy and menopause and result in discomfort or pain with vaginal intercourse ... Lubricating jelly....*

As if I don't know about this already. Sex, only one time since diagnosis, has just slipped further away.

Yesterday, on the phone, Johnny mentioned that he'd been married.

I tried not to sound too surprised. "Really?"

"It's not a topic I discuss at length."

"You don't have to tell me anything you don't want to."

"Neither of us wanted to get married or have kids," Johnny said.

"So?"

"Christine's parents were hard-line, old-school Catholics. They certainly didn't care much for me, which seemed strange that they would want me to marry their daughter. But it was all about 'religion.' Their marriage had been dead in the water for decades, but to get them off our backs—a pointless maneuver in retrospect—we did just that: no ceremony, all legalism, and later, the annulment.

"We'd lived together and been married for close to a decade and got along very well until Christine became bored, started hanging out with a bad crowd, and began doing methamphetamine which turned her into a monster within a few weeks. I couldn't even recognize her as the same person I had previously known and loved."

"Johnny, I'm so sorry."

One of the things I've always questioned about my brother is the company he chose to keep. But if you are imprinted with "you are useless and will never amount to anything," the people you might be drawn to could have serious problems of their own.

"I haven't seen her in years," Johnny said, then laughed. "We practiced tantra yoga."

"Ahh, great." What else could I say?

Unlike myself, it seems that he doesn't have many filters. We were raised in the same Catholic family where you didn't talk about sex. Taboos were laid down early. He'd overcome them. Good for you, Johnny. One less neurosis to deal with.

I keep thumbing through the *Guidebook.*

*"You may receive your transplant in the hospital and remain hospitalized until your blood counts recover, or you may receive your transplant in the*

*Cancer Center and remain under the care of the outpatient BMT team for approximately 100 days."*

I groan out loud. "One hundred days!"

I'd assumed two weeks, three at most. I read the paragraph again and heave the *Guidebook* across the kitchen floor.

# Chapter 49 - Full Freak Mode

THE FOLLOWING WEEK, I have an appointment at the Stanford Hospital for removal of my VAP and insertion of a Hickman Catheter. The Hickman allows blood to be taken and chemo administered without countless needle sticks in the chest as happens with the VAP. Sounds like a plus; but there are no illustrations of the Hickman in the patient handbook, so I'm not sure what I'm in for. The description in the *Guidebook* says:

*A central venous catheter is a soft flexible tube that is used to give medicine, fluids, blood transfusions, chemotherapy, or nutrition into a vein.*

Kind of vague. I don't think to Google it.

I ask the nurse who wheels me into the surgical suite about the anesthesia. She assures me that the conscious sedation will make the procedure painless and remove any memory of it. This turns out not to be true. I reckon that she (Stanford, in other words) might be ever so stingy with the feel-good drugs. I'd had a colonoscopy the year before at Kaiser and remembered zero except waking up in recovery where an angel of a nurse in a pearl necklace asked me if I wanted a cup of Pete's coffee, which I sorely did.

It's late on a Friday afternoon and two surgeons get to work. One of them removes my VAP while the other tackles the Hickman.

Insertion of the Hickman catheter requires two incisions, one at the jugular vein and another on the chest wall. At the jugular incision, also known as the "entrance" site, the surgeon creates a tunnel from the neck to the chest. Then the catheter is pushed through this tunnel. The exit site is where the tubes come out of the chest wall. The placement of the Hickman and removal of the

VAP hurts. A lot. And I remain alert during the whole procedure. I want to ask for more meds but decide to bear up and not be a baby. The two surgeons banter back and forth but neither speak to me. Okay, I can't repeat their exact words, but the jovial tone of their conversation makes me think they might slap each other on the back at any moment and say, "See you on the court in twenty. Loser pays for beers." I feel like nothing more than a collection of warm body parts on which a routine (for them) procedure must be completed before closing on a Friday. Going on for what seems like a long time, I am relieved when they finally finish sewing me up.

After the surgery, I get over my annoyance and tell the nurse that Dan and I are excited to be going out to dinner. Food restrictions more serious than those I had to adhere to during chemo will begin on Sunday—particularly with potentially high-microbial foods such as raw fish. I ask if I can have sushi, one last time for many months to come. "Sure," she says, "enjoy it."

Now, instead of the slight bulge of the VAP, I have two tubes sprouting from my chest a couple inches below my left collarbone. Honestly, being spared continual needle sticks will be a welcome relief, but the tubes emerging from me look and feel macabre. Still bald everywhere—yes, everywhere—the Hickman tubing pushes me into full freak mode.

Then we hit Friday evening traffic. It takes Dan nearly three hours to drive the sixty miles from Stanford to San Rafael through thunder, sleet, hail, and burned-out traffic lights. I come down off the measly amount of anesthesia shortly after our departure and suffer through the pain as we creep along. Sushi? What a joke. All I can do is to crawl into bed once we finally get home. Dinner never happens.

Placement of the catheter completes the first of two steps in my allogeneic conditioning preparing me for the main event, the stem cell transplant, aka, bone marrow transplant. Conditioning is such a pleasant, even tender, word and allogeneic has a ring similar to angelic.

# Chapter 50 - "Sugar, It's No Parade"

SUNDAY AFTERNOON, TWO DAYS after insertion of the Hickman, Dan and I blitz through a pile of paperwork at the Stanford Hospital Admissions Department. My fingers cramp; my lower back aches from standing. I can't read anymore and whatever I'm signing won't change what is about to begin anyway. Nearby, an orderly—wearing well-washed blue hospital scrubs, paper booties, and a surgeon's cap on his head—shifts his weight and strong-arms a wheelchair back and forth in anxious starts and stops.

Finally finished, I say to Dan, "There's nothing you can do here for the next six days. Go home and back to work."

"What if you need me?"

"I'll be fine." He lowers me into the wheelchair, and I whisper, "I love you. Go."

He kisses the side of my face. "Love you too. See you Saturday."

Saturday is my destination. I have no map. No itinerary. Just a paid transit to someplace I've never been and cannot imagine. I am the transplant.

As Dan walks away, I want to call out that I don't really mean it. *Stay with me, please.* Clutching the armrests of the wheelchair and biting my bottom lip, I blink and swallow to stop the tears. But I can't help it, they come. I watch until Dan turns a corner and is gone. He doesn't look back. The orderly wheels me away.

At home at Kaiser (odd that I now refer to Kaiser as "home"), I know my doctors and nurses, at least by sight. Dr. Arent, a.k.a., Big Bird, the handsome hospitalist, has always been so kind; the nurses (most), so skilled, and the aides, so helpful. The handsome food service fellow and the welcoming baristas at the espresso cart. These compassionate people are, of course, in addition to my irrepressible oncology cheerleader, Dr. Greyz. I have my dream team; and, with a couple of exceptions, it's great.

Here, I know no one. I am an anonymous middle-aged, female, bone marrow transplant patient clasping a small red duffle bag, which, like a lifeline, defines my real self—or more real self—not the medical record number, lab values, and data that will be the Stanford me for the next week. The canvas bag—containing a few toiletries, a bottle of the contraband sleeping pill Restoril, jeans, a black cashmere cardigan, and Barbara Kingsolver's *Poisonwood Bible*—says other things about me: I wear neutral colors, have insomnia, and appreciate good literature.

The orderly guides me and the chair to an elevator. We descend two stories from the ground floor and travel through hushed, dull gray hallways, the wheels click rhythmically, the orderly's paper booties scuff across the linoleum floor. It's Sunday evening and no one is around. I would have spoken to him, but my throat is too tight. What would I say? I'm scared to death and want to ask: *Can you rush me back out to the parking lot and stop my husband? Has anyone ever bolted?*

The *Guidebook* does not offer suggestions for appropriate conversational topics. I want to apologize for being distant; it's not like me. Nothing is.

We come to a set of double metal doors. He pushes a plate on the wall with his elbow. The doors open inward with a groaning whoosh, then clamp shut behind us. I startle at the metallic clap of those formidable doors. I've never been inside a jail or prison but imagine that the bolts and locks might sound the same.

Inside the sterile ward of blinking monitors and subdued lighting, nurses dart here and there but no one acknowledges us. The cool air is dry and thin, as if all the moisture has been sucked out of it. The nurses' station acts as a central hub and the patients' rooms form a wheel around it—a circular architecture that dispenses meta-medicine, scientifically beyond that provided in most hospitals. There are no plants or flowers. Microbes living on them could prove deadly. A stuffed bear holding a shiny mylar balloon is the only decoration. We wait. My jaw clenches.

A nurse notices us and says, "9A." Mine is the first bed as you enter room 9. The curtains are pulled between me and my roommates, revealing only the feet and lower legs of two other women already there. I grumble to myself but intimidation prevents me from asking for a private room. I also keep quiet because of a sense—however slight—of comradery. All of us are here to be transformed into someone new, and yet still who we were before we got sick. Forward and back. Time travel. Will it work? For some, yes; for others, no. Who can know the outcome?

Although we are sisters facing the same pain, and fear, and staggering odds, we don't speak to one another or even introduce ourselves. The question, "How are you?" would be senseless and crass. Except for occasional moaning, we are silent. There may be a lot of praying going on among the women in this ward.

That night I read *The Poisonwood Bible*, returning again and again to a favorite, dog-eared quote:

*"Sugar, it's no parade but you'll get down the street one way or another, so you'd just as well throw your shoulders back and pick up the pace."*

# Chapter 51 - Pretty in Pink

**DAY 1:** AFTER A DECENT NIGHT'S SLEEP, I am determined to throw my shoulders back and be Miss Congeniality of the Transplant Ward.

"Good morning," I greet today's orderly with a smile.

He nods and gestures to the wheelchair. I will get down that street, sitting or walking. I'm ready to pick up the pace and go wherever he takes me.

A nurse approaches. I greet her warmly as well.

"I have your HEPA."

"Sorry, what?"

"Your filtration mask. You can't leave the ward without it."

I frown as the nurse presents the transplant accessory. I'd never seen such a device, nor do I remember a description of it in the *Guidebook*; there were certainly no pictures. There was mention of a mask, but I imagined a small, delicate, paper cover-up in a pale yellow, the same that is worn by many people in Asian cities to avoid catching a cold or seasonal flu. The nurse demonstrates how to put it on and tightens it around my face. Made of a hard, gray rubber, the triangular-shaped mask covers my nose, mouth, and chin. Two large, bright-pink filters conceal my cheeks. The entire contraption has wide, adjustable straps that go around the top and back of my head to hold the monstrosity in place. With every anxious, artificial exhalation through those pink filters, my resolve to be a tough, model patient diminishes. The dangling tubes of the Hickman are strangely friendly, even comedic, compared to this bizarre HEPA guise.

I feel the hard rubber that obscures my face.

My awful, distasteful face.

During an awkward adolescence, my beautiful, heavy-lidded, tranquilizer-popping mother was aghast by my appearance. When I was thirteen and we stood in a Lucky supermarket checkout line, she scowled at me and said, "You used to be such a pretty girl. I don't know what happened to you."

Although I knew she was right, a slap across the face would have been far less painful. I much more resembled my dad's plain-Jane sister than my mother, and her disdainful, sideways glances never let me forget it. This was the same time that my dad had replaced me with Stacy. Both of my parents had now rejected me. In my homeliness, I'd become unwanted, disposable. This is the burden, the message I've carried since I stood in that supermarket line. It is how I still judge myself every time I pass a mirror or a window. I've hated photographs of myself and torn up a lot of them. When I was in high school, I was never asked on a date, or to a dance, so my mother was clearly right. And she despised me for my homeliness. Perhaps she felt angry that her daughter, who should have been a beauty, would turn out to be such a disappointment. What a sorry reflection on her!

With the HEPA covering my face, my mother's comment makes me burn all over again with anger and shame. I could have put the mask to good use back then.

My bald head protrudes from a blue flannel blanket wrapped around my shoulders, my feet are covered in brown hospital socks, and the damned HEPA respirator covers the bottom two-thirds of my face. At least in loose clothing, no one can see the tubes, but there is no hiding the freakish pink HEPA that defaces and consigns me to a sort of pathetic subspecies.

In silence, the orderly pushes the gargoyle me through a maze of underground hallways where the florescent lighting makes my hands appear lavender. I keep my eyes down as two hospital staff, then one visitor, pass by. At the radiology intake room, accessed by an unmarked door in an empty, obscure hallway, the orderly turns me over to a tech who wheels me into the heart of the subterranean department, a cold, shadowy space lit with only a few small spotlights in the ceiling. There are no windows in the black walls. Maybe because of the mask, there is no small talk between the tech and me.

When she asks me, "Can you stand?" I answer, *Yes*, but don't recognize my own voice.

The tech is sympathetic and relays instructions. Providing me with a block-like headrest, she removes my blanket and helps me lie on a table. A dark tangle of cables and camera-like devices festoon the ceiling. I lie still while she tattoos a permanent, small circle onto my chest that marks a central point for administration of the TLI.

From the *Guidebook:*

*Total Lymphoid Irradiation (TLI) is given to weaken your immune system to enable your donor's cells to grow. Immediate side effects are generally mild, but may include nausea, vomiting, decreased appetite, diarrhea, and fatigue. Other side effects that occur about a week later include a decrease in your blood cell counts. A decrease in blood counts places you at risk for infection, bleeding, and anemia. Late side effects of radiation include sterility, hypothyroidism and second malignancies.*

The tech leaves the room and sits behind a large pane of glass. The equipment in the ceiling moves and rotates with an efficient robotic sound. I am brought into the crosshairs of the radar gun. I am a bull's eye—or my immune system is—and administration of the radiation, while invisible and painless, forces me to lie motionless in a cold, dark room for what seems a long time. When finished, I wrap my flannel blanket around my shivering shoulders and wonder what Hades I have been dropped into. The same wordless orderly appears and wheels me back to the ward. I don't blame him for his silence. When I thank him for his help, my voice sounds as if I'm being strangled.

Back in the ward, my mask is removed and a nurse administers Anti-Thymocyte Globulin (ATG) into my Hickman. ATG—the second weapon used to wipe out an immune system—is repeated infusion of antibodies that prevent and, if necessary, treat rejection in bone marrow transplant patients.

Again and again, I return to my mantra, *Sugar, it's no parade....* It's the only thought that seems to help. Miss Congeniality has left the building.

I read the *Poisonwood Bible* all afternoon, going back again and again to a passage that most intrigues me:

*"I could never work out whether we were to view religion as a life insurance policy or a life sentence. I can understand a wrathful God who'd just as soon dangle us all from a hook. And I can understand a tender, unprejudiced Jesus. But I could never quite feature the two of them living in the same house. You wind up walking on eggshells, never knowing which ... is at home at the moment."*

I dangle from a hook. I walk on eggshells but to where, I don't know. I hope it is not a wrathful God, but a tender Jesus, who will determine what Johnny has to go through.

**Day 2:** I receive another cold 80cGy dose of radiation. This morning's radiation only lasts about thirty minutes and is more tolerable than yesterday's. Even though I feel like an anonymous freak, I cooperate and say please and thank you to everyone.

After I am returned to the ward, I receive the second dose of ATG.

"Day two can be tough," warns the nurse, "but some people have no problem. Hopefully, you'll be one of those."

Hours later, I moan. Shadows cross the doorway. There is so much shuffling. The nurse says my temp is 104; my body throbs, my hands and feet burn crimson. I beg for morphine, but don't know if they give it to me. I beg for ice but can't remember if I get that either. Like sandpaper, the sheets are unbearable. I must leave. Dan will take me home. The vast night is merciless. What is all that shuffling?

**Day 3:** The smell of oatmeal is revolting. More radiation. My temperature remains above 103. I writhe in bed. I want to scream, but don't know how. I haven't seen the sky in days. *Sugar, it's no parade.*

There is no tender Jesus in my house today. I beg a nurse to call Dan.

Except for a young Hispanic man who comes to visit the woman in the far bed by the window once a day, there are no other visitors to our room. I've never seen the woman behind the last flowered partition, but assume she is his mother. He doesn't look at me when he passes by. He goes to the woman and they pray. Our Father ... *Nuestro Padre.*

I wonder, *what can our Father do for them, for me, for any of us?*

Today, when the Hispanic man comes to visit and he and his mother begin to pray, I remember Elizabeth Targ, MD, a research psychiatrist I'd known professionally. She studied prayer and healing. Her research indicated that AIDS patients who were prayed for, often at a distance of thousands of miles, had better outcomes than those patients who were not prayed for. Most remarkably, the AIDS patients didn't know they were being prayed for, and yet their health improved.

In early 2000, Dr. Targ began to study patients with malignant gioblastoma multiforme, the most common and aggressive brain tumor in humans. This is the cancer that killed Senators Edward Kennedy and John McCain. Even with radiation and chemotherapy, median survival is fifteen months. Without treatment, it is four to five.

Dr. Targ was deeply involved in the study of remote healing and whether it could benefit these very sick GBM patients when she learned that she, herself, had gioblastoma multiforme. At announcement of this hideously bizarre twist of fate, a community of remote healers began to pray for her, and Elizabeth Targ received the very best care Western medicine could provide. Yet weeks short of her forty-first birthday—she died.

I don't believe that Elizabeth Targ ever gave up. She succumbed to a cancer so malevolent that no one, no prayerful intention, and no pharmaceutical or radiation could have done any more for her.

Gael has people praying for me, but I don't know how to pray anymore; I've forgotten the words. It's not like riding a bicycle. If I prayed, I'd feel like a fraud—only coming around and asking for help in my misery. Yet, I wonder if I should try.

In the evening, Dan arrives in a dark brown suit. He wears the required booties over his shoes and a paper mask on his face. I cry the moment I see him. Through the mask, he kisses the side of my face. He looks at my scarlet hands and murmurs, "Oh God."

I hide them in a fold of the blanket.

"I'm sorry to have called you."

"I should have been here before."

I love his face and body in this alien world. I grasp his sturdy arm. "I can't do this."

"You can."

"I'm disappearing."

Dan caresses the side of my face then lays his hand on my shoulder. "This is your big win, Honey. We've got to hold onto that."

"Do you think I should pray?"

He looks at me with widened eyes. "Why?"

"I don't know."

"Well, you know," he says, "I don't think there's a God behind the curtain meddling in our lives, if that's what you're asking."

"But it couldn't hurt, could it?"

"No, Honey. It couldn't hurt. But you are going to get well. I know that. God or no God."

"No dude behind the curtain?"

"No dude."

We smile at each other. I close my eyes. Sometime later I wake. Dan is gone.

**Day 4:** My fever is under 102 and the body aches are tolerable, but now there is something else—from my groin to my knees grows what resembles a purple mold. Does it give off a slightly sulfurous smell? More drugs are prescribed to address this painfully foul side effect.

After morning radiation, the nurse administers the day's infusion. I call Dan and tell him I am better. He doesn't need to come back.

Gael's tall votive still burns for me. If she were here, she'd be on her knees with my Hispanic neighbor. Some people, like Johnny's landlady Kathy, find it reassuring to think there are no accidents—that events are predetermined and happen for a reason due to an underlying order in life that dictates outcomes for each and every one of us. Yet there is no indisputable evidence of Fate or an involved God, kind or cruel. On the other hand, I approach these issues with a big dollop of humility. How can anyone know for certain, one way or the other?

**Day 5:** As my immune system diminishes, my isolation increases, and on Friday morning a nurse wheels me into a tiny private room. After the ATG and irradiation this week, most of my immune system is gone. While more immunologically fragile than ever, I surprisingly begin to feel better. I've finished the ATG, but the radiation will continue for several more days.

That evening, Elspeth; her best friend, Katie; and Katie's boyfriend, Mike, pay me a surprise visit. To enter my pint-sized room, they are required to don full surgical garb, including masks. I sport my pink respirator. Each of them comes in, wide-eyed and slowly as if they don't want to disturb anything, not even the air.

"I'm so embarrassed for you to see me in this." I point to the despicable HEPA.

"Oh Mom, it's okay."

"Please tell your dad about it. He's not seen it and I don't want to scare him when he picks me up tomorrow."

Elspeth is strong. She doesn't cry—at least not now—and acts as the graceful hostess while Katie never lacks for something sweet and charming to say. But the look of agony and wonder in Mike's eyes is a give-away; this is no easy visit for him. It is hot and claustrophobic in my tiny room. There are no chairs. Mike fidgets. While the conversation is light, even jovial, I encourage them to get on with their evening.

"I am smiling under this mask. You just can't tell," I say as my daughter leans in to kiss my forehead.

**Day 6:** I want out of this ward like I've never wanted anything before and on Saturday—so exhausted I don't know if I should laugh or cry—I am wheeled out of Stanford Hospital into a brilliant March morning. I haven't seen the sun, or sky, or outdoors in a week. For a brief reckless moment, I consider wrenching the HEPA off my face and sucking in a deep breath of real air.

I am unrecognizable in the mask, sunglasses, and a wool cap. My body is smaller than ever. I stand and Dan helps me stagger to the car. In the last six days, I've only walked a few steps to and from the bathroom and my legs are weak. My everything is weak, diminished, vulnerable. Yet I smile and move forward. To where, I don't know. My life is not my own. I must trust—in what or whom, I'm not sure.

Today, Dan and I will begin living as residents of the Oakwood in Mountain View, a large complex of corporate apartments a twenty-minute drive from Stanford Hospital and about seventy miles south of our home in San Rafael. Dan will be my around-the-clock caregiver for the next one hundred days. Back at home, we have help. A friend will housesit, take care of Harriet, and send us our mail. Laurie has generously offered to care for the ever-rewarding Spirit.

The Oakwood's lush and semitropical landscaping improves the appearance of the architecture, which bears a strong resemblance to college dormitories. It has outdoor pools and hot tubs, into which, of course, I cannot put so much as a toe. The Oakwood caters to two types of residents: corporate executives from around the world who have come to work in Silicon Valley for longer than they might want to stay in a hotel, and transplant patients from Stanford who look as I do with bald heads and pink respirators. The executives stride, the patients shuffle. I assume the Oakwood staff has warned the business clientele about us, in a compassionate, yet scientific-sounding, sort of way.

While still needing to rest most of the day, the symptoms I'd experienced in the hospital have lessened; my hands and feet only tingle and no longer burn. The purple mold growing down my thighs is shrinking.

Dan and Elspeth lug boxes up from the car while I watch from the couch. Our one-bedroom, one-bath apartment is furnished like a Holiday Inn, but there are two wide sliding glass doors that overlook the pools and the landscaping. The rooms are bright and airy. I tell myself that the worst is over. *I'm okay. Something new and better is coming.*

# Chapter 52 - How Could a Mother?

ON SUNDAY, DAN DRIVES ELSPETH to the San Francisco Airport for her flight back to L.A. and picks up Johnny who—once again—has been generously dropped off by Jeff and Kathy. Kaiser has paid for his own Oakwood apartment, decorated for a guy in stylish browns, tans, and charcoal.

Speaking of Kaiser, I am immensely grateful. They have done so much to save my life and my wallet and continue to pick up my enormous medical bill.

Cancer and money are not strange bedfellows.

Being in the medical education field, I've heard health economists say, with all due respect and disassociation: *Death is very cost effective.* A deceased patient is no longer a drain on health care resources. It's the treatment that's expensive. And as sad as it is, even in these wealthy United States, cancer can have a devastating monetary effect on victims and their families.

For some very unfortunate people, facing serious illness also means financial ruin. The gnawing message abrades: *This is going to cost a fortune.* How do people without insurance, or with inferior coverage, get access to quality health care? I can work myself up into a lather about the uninsured, or underinsured, woman who'd been diagnosed—as I—with stage 4 Mantle Cell Lymphoma. Without adequate insurance, without the very best treatment, her life is at stake. Her chances of survival: slim to none. I wonder what I would do. Would I use all of my resources for chemo, or spend every dime of my retirement savings for a bone marrow transplant—if I even had enough to pay for it? Could I ask my husband to sell our home for a treatment that had no guarantee of success? Would he insist? Or not? Just thinking about these questions makes my stomach churn.

It's daunting that uninsured, or underinsured, people who receive a devastating diagnosis must choose to become a pauper to simply have a shot at a remission. This is, of course, assuming that they have resources to sell. I get angry just thinking about this *Sophie's Choice* that some very ill people must face. In the United States, people like me in every way—except for their insurance coverage—are forced to make this wrenching decision or face the very real prospect of dying. What kind of an Effed-up situation is that?

DAN OPENS THE DOOR TO the trendy studio and Johnny stops. A crease forms between his eyebrows; he looks confused.

"Home sweet," I say and walk inside.

The air is warm and carries a faint floral scent of chemical cleaner, like an office or an airport, where lots of people have been but no one has ever lived.

Johnny enters. Seeing him in this apartment, I know with certainty that there is no turning back. The transplant will happen, and it could kill me or save me. The colors are muted. Perhaps the space is meant to soothe. It's a nice room. My brother's colorful tie-dye tee shirt is a paradox; he's a non sequitur in this room meant to house Silicon Valley executives. I doubt that this corporate enclave is a world he's ever walked into.

"You gonna be okay here?" I ask.

"Sure."

"If you need anything, you know where to find us."

On Monday, I continue to receive radiation, while Johnny begins his preparation for the transplant: two daily doses of Neupogen injections that will force his marrow to produce so many stem cells that they will crowd out of his bones and spill into his blood stream. Side effects of all this Neupogen include aching hip and leg bones and flu-like symptoms, but he doesn't complain. Every evening, Dan cooks dinner for us and drinks wine that neither

Johnny nor I can so much as sniff. But we have time to talk, and he tells me of the things that Bev did to him when us older kids were at school. How she berated him, made him feel unwanted and undeserving of even a shred of kindness. His traumatic experience being left on the swing set and losing consciousness. His retelling of abuse breaks my heart.

"How could a mother…?" I shake my head.

"The feeling of not measuring up," Johnny says, "the shame of being a poor performer, did remain as shadow material throughout my life. This intense feeling of inadequacy created the desire to keep my distance from all family members."

How tragically ironic that her most focused and brightest child would be the one who our mother would convince would never succeed.

"I've made peace with all that past turmoil. Nothing valuable or truly creative comes from self-pity. I engaged in that long enough to see its destructiveness, but it did take me years to set down the animosities I had toward Mom. One cannot expect love or compassion from someone living in hell."

The generosity of his comment stuns me. I cannot imagine how he has stayed as strong as he is. As kind. As serene. At that moment, I hate my mother, and my father, even if Johnny does not.

# Chapter 53 - The All-Day Sucker

JOHNNY'S TWICE-DAILY INJECTIONS continue, as does my radiation. On Thursday, he gets hooked up to an aphaeresis apparatus labeled the All-Day Sucker, Stanford's nod to humor. Blood is removed from his right arm and pumped into the All-Day Sucker where the heavier stem cells settle out. Then the lighter-weight blood is pumped back into his left arm. The Christ-like analogy of Johnny with his long hair, serene face, and needles in each arm, pinning him to the chair, is unavoidable.

The aphaeresis machine routes the stem cells—a stunning orange-coral color, like salmon roe—into a collection bag. Dan and I sit with Johnny and watch as the cells begin to swell the bag.

"They're gorgeous," I say.

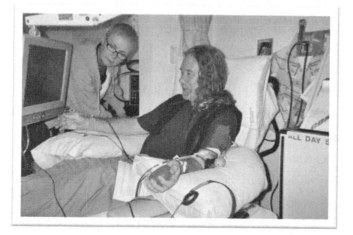

*Susan, Johnny, and The All-Day Sucker*

He smiles and relaxes in a spacious leather recliner while squeezing a large red sponge, shaped like a blood cell. Dan begins taking pictures. Johnny and I look like siblings, me hairless and more delicate, but the tribal resemblance is unmistakable.

The room is large, white, and filled with machinery that softly hums and warms the space. The three of us are alone and the mood in the room is private, even intimate.

Dan shows me a couple of photos he's taken and I hand the camera to Johnny. "Look at you, saving my life."

He clears his throat and looks down at his hands.

"You did so much for me, Sis."

"You deserved way more."

*What does he think I did for him?*

Did he know that for decades, I railed at Beverly about her cruel mistreatment of him? She would always respond with, "There's so much you don't know." But I understood from the beginning that something was very wrong between my parents.

I was eight years old. I'd been asleep when my mother woke me with her screaming, "Get off of me." I got out of bed and walked into the kitchen. My dad had her pinned down on the table and was standing between her legs, her dress pushed up around her hips. She saw me at the door and yelled, "Get me help. Go for the neighbors." But I couldn't move. I was too terrified and too ashamed. She begged me again, but I couldn't. Then my dad got off of her and growled, "Goddammit." She pushed her dress down. I was terrified when he walked past me and waited for a slap, but it didn't come. He smelled of liquor and cigarettes. My mother came into my bed that night. We never talked about what I'd seen. The thing I thought of the moment my mother pleaded with me to get the neighbors was how perfect their life looked. They were a young couple who had no kids. They had boxers, those beautiful dogs, a perfect dichondra lawn, and new cars. I was so ashamed of my family and of myself, as if this awful thing that had happened made me dirty and bad as well. I could never show them, or anyone, the ugliness that went on inside our house.

The memory of that night has never left me and, as I got older, it began to occur to me that Johnny might very well have been the result of spousal rape, or at least coerced intercourse, whatever the difference might be. Perhaps there had been many nights like that one. Still, I could never let my father's violent behavior excuse my mother's mistreatment of her own child. It was so monstrously unfair. As bad as my father was to her, Johnny never deserved the cruelty he suffered at her hands. Maybe I could understand her hating my father, but not Johnny, not her baby, not her little boy.

I never saw Beverly hug or kiss him or hold him in her lap. Read to him. She never smiled at him. When she spoke to Tom or Randy, her voice had a lilt. When she spoke to Johnny, her voice was clipped and flat, always bordering on anger. And tying him into his crib was unforgiveable.

Our animosity came to a head one day while I visited her in Los Angeles. I was thirty; it was two years before I got married. We stood in her bedroom.

*"Your brother was terrible," she said.*

*"I guess you mean Johnny."*

*"The way he talked to your grandfather and me was so disrespectful."*

*"And how did he get that way?"*

*"I know you blame me, but there is so much you don't know."*

*I left the room. I couldn't hear anymore.*

*"He hid drugs all over the house," she yelled while following me down the hallway.*

*"I really don't want to talk about this."*

*"You need to hear it. You need to know what I went through with him."*

*"Did you ever show him love or affection? I can't remember a single time. What do you think that kind of hatefulness does to a child?"*

*"Oh, you exaggerate so much," Beverly screamed.*

*Lacing up my tennis shoes, I yelled back, "I don't exaggerate anything."*

*"You will just never understand."*

*"I'm going out."*

*I opened the front door then slammed it behind me. I began to jog. I ran for miles, for well over an hour. On the way back to her house, I stopped at a florist and bought my mother flowers. I told her I was sorry and that it would never happen again. And it didn't. Over the next few years, she tried to bait me several times by bringing up all of the difficulties she'd endured with Johnny, but I'd change the subject or walk away. The end of our hostilities created a gaping emotional distance between us. Fighting is intimate. Detente is isolating.*

Johnny squeezes the spongy blood cell. The bag of stem cells slowly fills. I want to ask him what he means by *you did so much for me* but cannot go back to any more painful memories.

"It was nice of Jeff and Kathy to bring you down again."

"They're good people."

"I hope you don't mind me asking…."

"It's fine."

"Do they always drive you?"

"I don't drive."

"Why not?"

"I was maybe eight or nine and hit my head."

"I don't remember."

"I didn't tell anyone."

"What happened?"

"I was fooling around in the flood control behind our house and I slipped and hammered my head on the concrete. I think it knocked me out. I was pretty messed up."

"You never told Mom?"

"No, I was afraid she would hit me for being stupid." Johnny has a faraway look.

"God, Johnny."

"It's okay. I have no, or almost no, peripheral vision on the right."

"Oh."

"My bike's fine."

"But dangerous. You've already lost a tooth."

"No worries."

But the story does worry me. The lack of peripheral vision is another issue he's had to deal with. I sigh and glance at my watch. "You okay here?"

He nods.

"Dan and I have an appointment with a transplant nurse. I'm so sorry about the fall."

He smiles, clicks on the monitor over his recliner, and the film *A Beautiful Mind* comes onto the screen. He will be here another couple of hours donating stem cells for the transplant, possibly, hopefully, scheduled in the morning.

IT'S 9:00 AM, MARCH 24, 2006, my new birthday. It rained last night and the sky is translucent blue. Dan, Johnny, and I arrive at the Cancer Center. I am incognito in the HEPA, sunglasses, and my cap. Dan supports me as I still need help walking more than a couple minutes.

"You're trembling," he says.

"I'm excited."

We don't wait long before Andrea, a transplant nurse, escorts us through a set of heavy glass doors, beyond which I am allowed to remove the HEPA. We have been warned that one pass might not be enough and aphaeresis might need to be repeated. For Johnny's sake, I hope not.

We walk down a corridor with gleaming beige flooring and white walls toward a private room. Before entering, I see them from the hallway and cover my mouth with my hand. The smallish plastic bag of exquisite coral stem cells hangs on a metal tree next to the bedside. "Oh," escapes my lips. All four of us stand outside the room looking in.

"That is a miracle," I say.

"Made to order for you, Sis."

"I'm afraid to go in."

Dan leads me gently inside. "Your hands are freezing."

Andrea follows us into the room. Gesturing toward the bed, she says, "Please get comfortable." She takes my blood pressure, temperature, and several vials of blood. "Any pain?"

"No."

"You look wonderful," she says. "Would you like some music?"

"I'd love music."

She pulls a small CD player out of her bag. Indian flute music fills the room. I think of the lovely Meera. She must have had her transplant by now and might even be home.

Dr. Craig, my transplant specialist, joins us. Plump and in his late thirties, he has an impish face and is always smiling. He brims with optimism, and the confidence he instills in me is huge. I love this man. Being around him makes me believe that everything will be fine.

Dr. Craig hooks up the stem cells that begin to flow downward into my Hickman. I wear a pink sweater with a draped neck allowing the white Hickman tubing to fall down my chest. Dan takes photographs. My hair, no more than half an inch in length, covers my head in a soft mat. Johnny, in his tie-dye tee shirt, leans in toward me. Our smiles are irrepressible as the life-giving stem cells find their way to a new home.

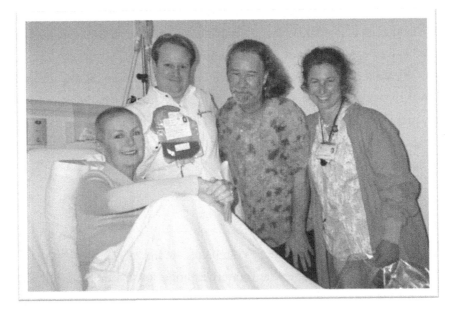

*Susan, Dr. Craig, Johnny, and Andrea*

"Feeling okay?" Dr. Craig asks.

"Great."

Johnny gives me a thumb's up.

Looking at the luminous orange bag, Dr. Craig says, "I believe this transplant will be your ticket to a cure and many more years of good health."

The other C word: *Cure.*

"You really think so? No one has said 'Cure' to me before."

"Yes, I really think so."

Tears run down my face. Dr. Craig leans over and hugs me. Dan tears up and hugs me; both of us are laughing and crying.

"This is the best news I've heard in the last six months. No, this is the best news I've ever heard. Thank you. Thank you so much." My voice is squeaky with emotion.

"Thank your brother, here."

"Yes, Johnny. You are literally a life saver."

We hug and his long hair covers both of us as if we are in a secret society where only those who share blood and bone are admitted. His stem cells— like microscopic homing pigeons on a life-and-death mission—are on their way into my bone marrow to set up house. If all goes well, these cells will destroy any cancer still hiding in my body and give me a new, nonmalignant immune system and the promise of years of health to come.


THAT EVENING OVER DINNER at our tiny kitchen table, I ask Johnny, "Have you seen a doctor about your vision?"

"It was a long time ago."

"I can help you get it checked out."

He shrugs. *Does that mean no?*

"It was amazing, wasn't it, how I found you? That ZabaSearch thing."

"Yeah." he nods. "It was lucky."

"I was surprised your number was listed."

"It had been unlisted for a very long time, but then I started getting crank calls."

I lean toward him. "When?"

"A couple months back. I got my number changed and told the phone company to keep the new number unlisted, but they didn't."

"Wait a minute," says Dan, now also leaning in toward Johnny.

"What a mistake, huh?" says Johnny.

"You had an unlisted number for…" Dan continues.

"Over ten years." Johnny finishes the sentence.

"You start getting crank calls and request another unlisted number?" I ask.

"Yeah. Somebody screwed up."

"So, for a very brief period of time, your number got listed?" I feel myself staring at him, forehead creased, incredulous.

"It might have been a week before I found out my number was listed."

"Are you saying that during one particular week, my friend Anne does a search and finds you?" I ask.

Nodding his head, Johnny gazes intently into my face.

"So, if Anne would have looked a week before or a week after, I wouldn't have found you?"

"I guess something like that."

"A mindless clerical error saved my life?"

"You could look at it that way," says Johnny.

"Good God."

Dan takes a long swig of wine. I stir the macaroni and cheese on my plate and feel something I can only describe as wonder. Was there someone or something behind the curtain when that little screw-up happened?

Although he doesn't say so, I sense that Johnny is anxious to leave the Oakwood and get home to his geckos, chickens, and marijuana plants. The next morning, Dan and Johnny accompany me to Stanford for my daily visit to the BMT Clinic. At the clinic door, Johnny gives me a long, affectionate hug.

"I'm glad to be getting back home, but I'm happy I was able to help."

"You are heroic, Johnny."

"That's way too big a word. But having accomplished something for you suits me just fine."

"I'll never forget what you've done for me."

"I love you, Sis."

"I love you too."

I wave goodbye as he and Dan leave, on their way to the San Francisco Airport where Jeff and Kathy wait to drive Johnny back to Willits.

# Chapter 54 - Like a Therapist's Office or an Electrolysis Suite

WHILE MY BONE MARROW DOES the heavy lifting, my battles now are against fatigue and boredom.

On a typical day, we awake before 7 AM. I make a pot of coffee and Dan preps breakfast, usually cereal with no fresh fruit, or well-cooked eggs and toast. After breakfast, he wraps my chest with plastic and tape so I can shower without getting the adorable, two-tubed Hickman wet. I dress, wrestle the HEPA over my head, and Dan drives us to Stanford.

All of us respirator-wearing transplant patients are accompanied by a caregiver. We cannot travel alone. Some of us might wear slacks instead of sweats. Some of us cover our bald heads. Waiting in the reception area, I wonder how the other patients look without the masks, what they do, where they live. Who would make it, and who wouldn't? The clinic reception area has an atmosphere of privacy—almost shame—like a therapist's office or an electrolysis suite and doesn't invite conversation any more than the respirators do. Friendships are not forged in the waiting room—even the caregivers rarely converse.

Inside the clinic proper—which is isolated from the outside world with the heavy metal doors and where we can remove our HEPAs—the routine never varies: my weight is checked, my blood pressure and heart rate measured, and numerous vials of blood are drawn from the Hickman. I am then parked inside a private room to wait in bed all morning for the results of the blood tests. Dan works. With my limited energy and difficulty concentrating, I keep one or two simple work projects going that I can do from bed on my laptop. If my cell counts are okay, I am released to return the next day and do it all over again. Back at the Oakwood apartment, exhausted by the morning routine and barely able to hold my head up, I spend a couple hours napping—something I haven't done since I was a child.

During these long, tiresome days of recuperation, transplant guidelines prohibit me from cooking, cleaning, doing laundry, driving, exercising, or having sex. Dan has to do all of this; well, except for the sex part (I guess). He doesn't reach for me. I don't blame him. My body is alien to me and I imagine to him. We've had sex only once in the past eight months. But since I am bald, have no energy, and rubber tubes dangle from my chest, getting frisky in bed never makes the To-Do List. It's not that I like this dry spell but can do nothing about it beyond feeling bad for Dan and about as sexy as a HEPA filter.

Food choices are strictly limited and exceedingly boring. Still no alcohol, of course. Every drop of water I drink (the guideline is three liters a day) has to be boiled; and Dan does this generously and without complaint for one hundred days. No raw fruits or vegetables. No salad. No take-out, delivery, to-go, or otherwise pre-prepared food. And no pepper. Having seen the spice markets in India where huge piles of pepper in outdoor carts swarmed with thousands of flies, I understand this.

While we have a housecleaning crew once a week, Dan does all of the cooking (really), the grocery shopping, the dishes, and the laundry. So how can I be so crass as to even whisper that his cooking might have been the slightest bit dismal? I feel like one ungrateful slug to just think it. Even Dan would be the first to admit that cooking day-in and day-out is not his thing. Super helpful with anything around the house and always cheerful about pitching in, when it comes to cooking for more than a couple of meals in a row, his inspiration and energy for the task become as flaccid as the week-old red leaf lettuce in the refrigerator, which I can't eat anyway. A typical dinner consists of pasta (gluey) with a canned sauce and some overcooked vegetables. Lordy, I get tired of it. I gently suggest a cookbook, but he declines, stating that anything requiring more than four ingredients or three steps is too much work. I don't have a leg to stand on, so to speak, and really try to be grateful about the heaps of gummy pasta he presents many nights. However, desserts are allowed and boy do we indulge.

Today, there's good news: in just under a month, another bone marrow biopsy reveals that more than fifty percent of my marrow now comes from Johnny. The graft is taking, and we celebrate. We drive to Baskin-Robbins and Dan goes inside to buy a quart of butter pecan ice cream while I wait in the car and call Johnny with the news. When he gets back, we wolf down the quart as unconcerned about calories as gangly adolescents.

The end of chemo and radiation, and the return of an appetite, also means the end of being lean and bald. My hair begins to grow back. Andi McDowell? Not so much. Roseanne Roseannadanna is closer to the truth. Brillo pad-like hair sprouts from my scalp. And, with a diet of pasta, desserts, and no exercise, I start to pack on the pounds. Food tastes like food again. For lunch, I might have a tuna and mayonnaise sandwich with two pieces of bread—one piece of bread replacing the lettuce—and a cookie replacing the apple that I still can't have. Potato chips? Why not? On one visit with a Stanford oncologist, somewhere near the midpoint of our quarantine, I complain about gaining weight. Without much of a bedside manner, the oncologist looks at me as if I am insane, to which I say, "I guess I'm lucky to be alive." The empathetic doctor rolls her eyes and shakes her head.

In addition to everything else, my heroic husband takes on the daily flushing and twice weekly cleaning of the Hickman catheter. As a precision mechanical sort of job, it requires meticulous attention to detail, one of Dan's strong suits. He can tell you how anything is put together. Instructions for flushing and cleaning the contraption run on for five, single-spaced pages in the transplant guidebook. This daunting amount of instruction doesn't alarm him in the least, and he does an outstanding job at keeping my Hickman squeaky clean and operational for all the months I had it. That alone should win him the gold medal in caretaking.

In sickness and in health, baby. Despite no sex, Dan and I have never been so married.

# Chapter 55 - A Major Pain-in-the-Ass Troublemaker

EVERY FEW WEEKS, I am subjected to another bone marrow biopsy (BMB) to determine the progress of my transplant. The fourth one today rates as a calamity. Because Stanford is a teaching hospital, and the Fellows are on a rotation system, bone marrow transplant patients never receive a biopsy from the same physician twice. I feel thrown under the biopsy bus and believe that many of the Post-Doc Fellows need additional practice—Dr. Craig (who performed my third BMB) being the rare exception. Bone marrow transplant patients provide these young doctors with "opportunities for learning."

As an institution, Stanford has no protocol for these biopsies except that they be performed under local anesthesia, the same as Kaiser.

Today, the Fellow comes at me like a locomotive and seems to know nothing about the proper way to administer anesthesia in small, shallow sticks before plunging the entire syringe into my hip. (He's not the only one who uses this painful approach, but after my third biopsy by Dr. Craig, I realize that there is a right and a very wrong way to do this.) The ham-handed way the Fellow administers the anesthesia literally shakes me. I tremble on the table. When he inserts the boring needle, he can't get a sample. He pushes, reinserts at a different angle, and pushes some more. Finally, he mumbles, "Your right hip may be too scarred to yield any marrow."

*Oh great, he's going to have to start over on the other side.*

The intense pressure in my hip goes on and on, but he finally gets the right angle that releases the marrow and bone chip he's after. This guy must have been absent the day they taught BMB in med school. The experience is so grueling that it makes me determined to take on this misguided policy of nothing but local anesthesia. It's heartless that cancer patients should suffer repeatedly like this.

So, with the help of the Stanford medical librarian, I begin researching which healthcare facilities in the U.S. offer their patients "conscious sedation" for bone marrow biopsies and which do not. Conscious sedation (CS) can be achieved with a number of drugs, but the two most popular are fentanyl and versed.

Versed, a short-acting benzodiazepine (an example of a benzodiazepine is Valium) was developed in the mid-1970s and is used for inducing sedation and amnesia before medical procedures, among other indications. Versed enables the patient to be conscious during the procedure, such as a colonoscopy or certain oral surgeries, yet remember nothing of it. Really rather miraculous. Versed does decrease respiratory rate in about one quarter of patients and induce apnea in another fifteen percent, but studies report that these responses are transitory and have not been serious. Fentanyl is a potent, synthetic opioid analgesic (pain reliever) with a rapid onset and short duration of action. Quick in, quick out. It is not an error to classify these as happy drugs; perhaps that is why they are so hard to get.

While I admit that many of the institutions I contact in my little research project do not offer their biopsy patients this CS courtesy, many do. With completion of my data collection, I compose this letter to the current chief of staff. Oddly enough, he and I had been undergrads together at U.C. Berkeley, but the coincidence of our shared student years did nothing to further my cause.

*June 9, 2006*
*XX, MD, Division Chief*
*Professor of Medicine*
*Stanford University Medical Center*
*Division of Blood & Marrow Transplantation*
*300 Pasteur Drive*
*Stanford, CA 94305*

*Dear Dr. X:*

*My name is Susan Keller, and I am a patient at both Stanford Cancer Center and at Kaiser Permanente. I would first like to say that the care I've received, overall, at Stanford has been exemplary. The nurses have been especially kind, proficient, and helpful. I am also deeply grateful to my insurer, Kaiser Permanente, for the chemotherapy phase of my treatment as well as for their continuing financial support. Without them, I would not be where I am today. And where I am today is nine months post diagnosis from stage 4 Mantle Cell Lymphoma.*

*I received a non-myeloablative allogeneic transplant on March 24, 2006. [Blah. Blah. Blah.]*

*I am writing to you to ask that the Stanford policy of only local anesthetic for bone marrow biopsies and aspirations be revisited. [Blah. Blah. Blah.]*

*All facilities that I contacted will offer conscious sedation for BMBA, if requested. [Blah. Blah. Blah.]*

*I am attaching the written responses I got to my question. Here, in summary, is what I found: [Blah. Blah. Blah.]*

*No doubt a person could go on and on tallying up what happens where. I believe that the larger point is that the quick asleep, quick awake medications that are used universally for procedures such as endoscopy should be made available to those patients who must regularly endure painful procedures such as BMBA.*

*Another aspect of BMBA at Stanford is that the patient never knows who is going to perform the procedure. [Blah. Blah. Blah.]*

*I'm also enclosing a few abstracts on the subject. [Blah. Blah. Blah.]*

*Obviously, there is a financial aspect to changing policy, and clearly a local is less expensive than CS. [Blah. Blah. Blah.]*

*Thank you for your time in reviewing these materials. I look forward to hearing from you.*

*Sincerely,*

*Susan Keller*

*Enclosures*

I'll bet he rankled that I brought up anything to do with money. I can imagine him shaking his head and tut-tutting. Lit abstracts, how absurd, and from a *patient*. I'd printed out literature abstracts for other docs and they'd eyed them as if the papers might contain Ebola. But likely worst of all, he may have found the letter from the Mayo Clinic to be nothing short of insulting. I've seen physicians become defensive real fast when being told how someone else might do something different or better than they do. Dr. X probably labeled me as a major pain-in-the-ass troublemaker and a whiner and thought in a most superior way: "A little bit of knowledge is a dangerous thing."

While the letter, abstracts, and statement from the Mayo Clinic get me nowhere in terms of changing the Stanford policy on conscious sedation, with a lot of hollering, I get 2 mg of Valium (a very low dose) to relax me and fentanyl to help with the pain for my next, and fifth, biopsy. The fentanyl comes in a sucker, like a See's Candies caramel. Come on, why aren't all patients offered this small consideration, even if it is a placebo-sized dose? I'd like the Stanford staffers who do not allow conscious sedation to undergo a string of bone marrow biopsies themselves—from their occasionally inept Fellows—to physically experience their stingy and misguided policy. With the valium and fentanyl, I tolerate this fifth biopsy better than the previous one, and the Fellow who performs it seems to have attended class the day they demonstrated how it is done.

# Chapter 56 - Afraid of the Avian Flu?

"I ADVISE AGAINST IT, but if you must go, stay away from crowds."

Seven weeks' post-transplant, Dan and I take a gamble and, against the finger shaking of the Stanford Fellow, drive to Los Angeles to attend Elspeth's USC graduation.

The caution against crowds—and the infections they carry—becomes immediately laughable as we cram onto campus with no fewer than fifty thousand other parents, well-wishers, and students to listen to Mayor Antonio Villaraigosa deliver the commencement address to the overheated audience. Even in my horrid HEPA—looking as though I might not survive the mayor's remarks—no one offers me a seat, or even a planter box or window ledge to lean on. Dan and I stand for the achingly long speech of which I remember nothing except my desperate need to collapse. My head swelters under my wig. I think about bolting but have no idea where I would go or how I would get there through the throngs of thousands. After the commencement address concludes—and to my immense relief—all fifty thousand participants split off into smaller groups to attend their students' individual schools' ceremonies. For Elspeth's drama and journalism school graduation there are seats—thank God—in the air-conditioned Bing Theatre, a lovely old brick building covered in ivy. Michael, a close childhood friend of Elspeth's, also graduating, catches a glimpse of me in the audience. He knows I've been sick but hasn't had the pleasure of seeing me in my sterile regalia. A momentary look of alarm passes over his face until he realizes that I am the bizarre creature dolled up in a Martha Stewart wig and the freaky pink HEPA. His face falls, his eyes widen, and he appears stricken. After the ceremony, he hugs me for a very long time, my HEPA buried in his chest.

As we leave the Bing and walk toward the car to return to our motel so I can rest, we pass one of Elspeth's classmates and exchange a quick hello. We congratulate him and his family. Then his father turns to me and pointing to the mask says with a laugh, "Afraid of the Avian flu?" I also try to laugh (what comes out of my Darth Vader face plate sounds more like a snore or a snort) and say, "No, I wear it for other reasons."

We walk away. In a quick second, Elspeth receives a text from her friend deeply apologizing for the catastrophe of the comment. *"What a douche!" he says.* His father, as it turns out, is a physician. I laugh and feel sorrier for the oafish MD than for myself.

After the exertion of the morning, I need to lie down so badly I could have caved in right there on the USC lawn. We'd paid so much for tuition that I feel I own a piece of the campus anyway—why not the shady bit of grass here in front of me? Elspeth insists on coming back to the motel with us. I try to convince her to join friends for some post-college partying, but she refuses. Dan and Elspeth support me back to the car.

Our motel is on Highland, just south of the Hollywood Bowl. A river of cars surges past our windows full of fun-seekers on their way to the Southern California beaches, the varied delights of the Sunset Strip, or Disneyland, the Magic Kingdom.

We close the blinds and the brown room becomes gloomy; but despite the cheesy surroundings, I feel a joyful sense of completion and pride. My daughter has just graduated from a prestigious university with academic honors, and I am here to celebrate. A few months ago, my being alive at this time had been in question.

I lie down with Elspeth in one queen bed while Dan takes the other. Both of them fall asleep quickly while I watch their relaxed faces and smile. I remember sleeping with Elspeth when she was an infant and a child. I'd wrap my body around my girl's small, warm limbs. Her fuzzy blond head rested against my chest. Her steady breathing made me love her more than I thought possible. Now, as I rest my arm on my daughter's shoulder and feel her body gently rise with each breath, I am ransacked with emotion. I cannot bring that little girl back. The passage of time is cruel.

I look at the gold honor cords lying on the small writing desk along with Elspeth's graduation cap and gown and remember a day, maybe a year ago, when I walked through a department store and passed by the girls' dresses. My breath caught in my throat as I thought about how much, as a twelve-year-old, Elspeth would have loved these dresses, especially the one of pink taffeta and black velvet. Overcome with a feeling of emptiness and loss, my eyes stung. I stopped to touch the fabric and was struck by the pain of never being able to go back. All that was lost. That little girl, that preteen who loved to dress up, she was gone. Lying here now, I could sob at that memory. But wait. My daughter's shoulder rises. She is here. We have this moment. It is enough. It is everything.

I wouldn't have missed the graduation for anything but have never been as fatigued as when we get back to the Oakwood. Leaning on Dan, I can barely walk the few yards to our apartment. Dan helps me undress. Once in bed, I don't move for fifteen hours.

Two days later, back at the clinic, results of my blood work have the on-call doctor looking at me sideways and telling me that my kidneys have suffered from the trip. The setback is probably temporary, but there is an "I told you so" in his delivery. I doubt that he would miss his child's college graduation. The nurses dump bags of hydration through my catheter, and I return to drinking my three plus liters of water per day, all thoughtfully boiled by my loving, diligent, and devoted husband. It takes me a week to regain the paltry amount of energy I'd had before the trip. But it was so worth it.

# Chapter 57 - Aloha Is Hello and Goodbye

NO SEX; BOREDOM; BLAND, OVERCOOKED food; house arrest except for being a morning captive of the BMT Clinic: these describe the first two months post-transplant. Results of my last biopsy show that eighty-five percent of my bone marrow now comes from Johnny. I call to tell him of our progress.

He says, "I love you, Sis."

"I love you too."

The days close in on one hundred, a critical, post-transplant marker. Half of all BMT patients wind up back in the hospital. I don't. The seemingly eternal weakness and aches mean that my body is producing a new, nonmalignant immune system: The Holy Grail for all bone marrow transplant patients. Despite the daily malaise and headaches, I experience no serious complications until sharp, shooting pains on my right side begin, followed by a red rash containing small clear blisters from my hip to knee. It's an outbreak of the human herpes virus type 3 (HHV-3) that causes chickenpox in young people and herpes zoster (shingles) in adults. In transplant patients, it can spread to the lungs and become serious, even fatal. My HHV-3 virus receives immediate attention, and I am prescribed an IV drip of acyclovir. To accomplish an around-the-clock drip without admitting me to the hospital, I'm given an IV shoulder bag—like a backpack—that feeds into my catheter. The nurses teach Dan how to draw acyclovir (the shingles med) from vials and inject it with a sizable hypodermic syringe into the bag in a sterile manner. Now, in addition to the tubes protruding from my chest and the pink HEPA, I lug around a heavy backpack of medicine; and Dan adds a new skill to his growing medical CV.

I don't (often) allow myself to go to the dark place—*these blisters could do me in*. That's ridiculous. I've been through much worse and can handle the pain. I'm a tough traveler of the transplant journey. I've carried a lot, much more than a sloshing daypack.

As I hobble down the clinic hallway, Arjun—Meera's husband who I'd met at the Transplant Orientation Class—walks toward me while gazing at the floor. His guileless, even childlike face that was charming with laugh lines around his eyes, has changed. His straight back—that gave him an air of confidence, as if he shared his wife's optimism that she, and everyone else cared for at Stanford, would be just fine—is now slumped. His previous vitality appears to have been wrung out of him.

"Arjun?"

He looks up. His expression is blank and disoriented, as if I'd just woken him.

"Yes?"

"I'm Susan. We met at Orientation. Isn't Meera through with all of this?"

"No."

"Wasn't she ready for transplant?"

"She can't be transplanted."

"What?" I am stunned and alarmed. "Her brother's a perfect match."

He glances away then back at me.

"She can't sustain a remission."

"Oh, no. I'm so sorry."

"How are you?"

"Okay. Except for this." I say, pointing to the backpack.

"Is it serious?"

"No."

He nods, takes a couple steps, then turns, "Best of luck to you."

The next day, I ask my nurse about Meera. She shakes her head, "Not good. Room 103."

Making my slow, painful way toward Meera's room, I question my motivation with every step. I feel voyeuristic inserting myself into this family's private moment. Still, I want to speak with her. The door is ajar. As I'm about to knock, a doctor approaches.

"You can't go in."

"What?"

"Your shingles."

"But…"

"You can't," he says and hurries away.

Keeping me in the hallway is stupid—my shingles are not a threat to Meera—but arguing outside of a dying woman's room is senseless and rude. I tap on the door.

"Come in," says a girl.

I push the door open but remain where I am. Stephanie, Meera's daughter, cradles her mother in bed. Her arms wrap around Meera's bird-like body. Stephanie's hair is tangled and her eyes are red. Arjun sits at the bedside holding Meera's hand. He looks exhausted and distant. His khaki slacks and brown polo shirt are the same he'd worn the day before. Meera's dark hair frames her tiny face like an ebony halo against the pale-blue pillow. She looks so small, smaller than her twelve-year-old daughter.

Taking a half step into the room, I breathe in the scent of curry and onion—a savory aroma I'd not smelled in months. White Styrofoam takeout containers—full of chicken, rice, and red lentils—are piled up on a bedside table. The smells make me hungry but I'm ashamed of myself for thinking about food.

The room is silent: no labored breathing or whimpers of pain. The monitors have been removed. No beeping machinery. No music, just the heavy hush of sorrow and resignation. Standing in the doorway with my hands in fists, the muscles of my face are tight while I push back the tears. I am an intruder. My obvious good luck makes me feel guilty; I want to apologize or leave, but don't.

"Mom," says Stephanie.

Meera opens her eyes, looks at me, and raises her fingers gracefully off the bed like a gesture of aloha, saying both hello and goodbye.

"Sorry. They won't let me come in."

The three of them gaze back at me with wan smiles.

"Meera, you are a wonderful woman. You helped me so much. At the beginning."

I swallow against the growing lump in my throat and continue.

"Everything about that orientation was so frightening until I met you. I felt better just being in the same room with you. You called me a Smarty Pants and we both laughed. Remember?"

Meera nods.

"She appreciates hearing that," says Arjun.

"Give her a kiss from me," I say to Stephanie.

"Thank you for coming by," says Arjun.

"I'll be thinking of all of you."

Stephanie kisses her and Meera closes her eyes.

Walking back to my room, tears slide down my face. I cry for Meera, Arjun, and Stephanie, but also for myself, for Dan, and for Elspeth. I wonder, *Why Meera and not me? Could it still be me? Nothing is certain.*

I remember my conviction at diagnosis and throughout most of chemo and the transplant—*I will live. Death is not an option.*

I'm sure Meera felt the same, but she dies that night.

A week later, the shingles are gone and I'm done with the backpack.

# Chapter 58 - "I Mean Go. Go Home."

"YOUR HICKMAN IS GOING to be removed, so just stay put."

Not keen on being messed with anymore—I've just had another bone marrow biopsy, number six, and my back aches—the nurse's unexpected announcement surprises me.

Ninety-two days after insertion of the catheter, it seems that I'm going to say goodbye to my secret freaky friend. It's saved me dozens, if not hundreds, of needle sticks; it's given Dan another caregiving activity in which he excelled; and, while weird, I can keep it covered up. I have no problem with loose clothing. I will, though, be glad not to have to be wrapped up in saran to take a shower.

"Today? Now?" I ask.

"Yes. Then you are free to go."

I must have had a quizzical expression.

"I mean go. Go home. You are done with Clinic. Your care will be transferred back to your Kaiser oncologist."

"She has another week," says Dan.

"No. Her numbers are okay. She can go."

And so, like that, I am told that Stanford is done with me. No fanfare, no going-away party, I am free—an equally terrifying and exhilarating thought. Even though I've kvetched about some of the Stanford policies— especially their stinginess with feel-good drugs—the compassionate transplant champions have been at my bedside for nearly one hundred days. I've become accustomed to and trust the clinic routine. I feel safe and supported. Other people have had the answers. Tomorrow it will be me and Dan. Tomorrow I'm supposed to turn back into the woman I was before the lymphoma. But that woman is gone, and my replacement has not yet arrived. *Where is she? Will I recognize her? When might she show up? What will I do until she does?*

"Thank God," I whimper into Dan's shoulder. "I think."

Within a few minutes, a nurse practitioner (NP), small, slender, and about my age, arrives to wrestle with the Hickman.

"I can't believe this is the end of the road," I say.

"Well, not entirely. We'll have you back here for regular checkups."

"I'm actually glad to hear that."

The NP smiles. "We aren't going to toss you out just yet."

"But the days of the Hickman are over?" I ask.

She nods.

"So, how do you remove it?"

"I just yank." Her straightforwardness strikes me as sarcastic or entirely graceless.

"That's it? You just yank?"

"Yup."

How, I wonder, after the long and complicated insertion process, can she just yank out the whole contraption without so much as a scalpel and some stitches?

"Sometimes I get the whole catheter and sometimes I only get the tubes. It's about fifty-fifty."

Dan's brow furrows as he stares at the NP.

"If I don't get it all, and you want the mechanism out, you'll have to have it surgically removed."

"If you don't get it, can it stay in there?" I ask.

"Oh, sure. It'll just be a little bumpy."

I look at Dan and shake my head.

"Ready?" asks the NP.

"I guess."

Standing directly over me with a bony left shin resting against my rib cage for leverage and both petite hands firmly clutching the base of the Hickman, the NP takes in a deep breath, and with an unceremonious grunt tugs mightily at the tubing. It's over before I feel any pain.

"Hmm," she says looking at the dangling tubes. Then she drops a ten-pound sandbag onto my chest.

"You will need to keep that there while the hole in your vena cava clots over."

"So, the rest of the Hickman is still in there?"

"Yeah, but it really doesn't matter that much."

I wonder if she would want one of these gizmos residing in her chest.

"It won't get infected or show up in airport security?"

"No."

"When my nephew broke his ankle, they had to put a screw in to hold it together; but a couple of years later, the screw started working its way back out."

"That won't happen. I guarantee it."

"Okay," I say, glad to have a chest that, while lumpy, does not make me look like a robotic alien.

With this last "medical intervention," we have "graduated" and are released from the confines of the Stanford Advanced Cancer Center. I can largely dispense with the HEPA and eat at restaurants. "House arrest" in Mountain View has ended and tomorrow we'll go home. As we walk out, I say goodbye to a couple of nurses who wish me the best; overall it is an entirely nonchalant exit, as if I'd just dropped by for an annual physical.

COMPARED TO THE TINY ONE-BEDROOM Oakwood apartment, our 2,600-square-foot rancher seems vast. Walking from room to room, I shake my head and whisper, "Thank you."

In the living room, I stop and look at our front door. I think about Stephanie and Arjun. What did they feel the first time they walked through their front door without Meera? It must have been a very hollow pain. There will always be an emptiness in their home, the shape and size, and warmth of their beloved Meera. How am I home while she is not?

Even though fatigued, I do what I always do after being away from home for more than a few days—I pull the broom from the closet and begin to sweep.

"Honey," Dan says, "the house has just been cleaned. I made sure of that."

"It's not about dust. I'm reconnecting."

But he knows this. He's seen me sweep dozens of times; he bought me the sturdy broom and painted exotic-looking eyes on the front of it. Pushing the stiff bristles across the broad wooden planks soothes me. Moving through my bright kitchen, I have a sense of completion, of reward, of assurance that all will be well. I am home. I am happy. I dare to say, I am healthy.

I fall in love with our wool rugs, linens, and spice drawers, I'm eager to make the bed, shop for groceries, fold clean laundry. I begin to cook again, delighting in the recipes from my collection of cookbooks: seared salmon with lime, maple syrup, and siracha; fingerling red potatoes baked in parchment with garlic and rosemary; Thai curry. Salads with little gem lettuces, radicchio, and arugula. Raw fruit. Pepper is now okay. Wine too.

Dan returns to work.

As the doses of immunosuppressant drugs decrease, my strength comes back. The headaches lessen. I take on more work projects. My current challenge, particularly without the HEPA, is to stay disease and microbe free. Any medical office or hospital visit requires the respirator. I must avoid crowds, public transit, and those who are sick. Also, as my platelet counts are still extremely low, internal bleeding remains an issue. I see Dr. Greyz frequently and have blood tests every few days.

I ask her, "What is the greatest threat I face?"

She doesn't hesitate. "The lymphoma coming back."

*No.* That is behind me, as if the cancer happened to someone else. I'll not look over my shoulder as if stalked by disaster. My view is forward. Only forward.

# Chapter 59 - An Eating Machine with a Loathsome Attitude

I'VE BEEN HOME FOUR MONTHS and have just checked the computer for results of my blood test today. My liver function tests—indicators of liver injury—panic me. They are more than twenty times normal. Is this a meltdown? The Chernobyl of my liver? Three Mile Island?

It's after 7 PM. I leave an urgent phone message for the on-call oncologist at Stanford and wait. I pace and wonder if I should be in an ambulance or checking into the ER. I phone Gael and ask her what to do. She demurs, "I hardly have a thumbnail of information about liver function; in fact, I barely have a hangnail of knowledge."

I laugh out loud. "Well, if my liver gives out while we're on the phone, I will have died laughing."

Dan wants to take me to the hospital but I convince him to wait until we hear from Stanford. Getting a call back, the oncologist assures me I'm not dying on the spot but must go to Kaiser tomorrow for more testing.

After blood work the next day, I get the diagnosis: Chronic Graft versus Host Disease (GVHD), a disorder that commonly develops in donor-transplant patients after day 100. Twelve to fifteen percent of patients die from Chronic GVHD, not the most terrifying odds. I'd faced much worse and gone way too far to be knocked down now.

Along with the alarming liver counts, white, lacy oral ulcerations cover the inside of my mouth, another sure sign of GVHD. Treatment is Prednisone.

Prednisone is used for a huge variety of illnesses and disorders, and—almost miraculously—cures or greatly improves many dire and more mundane conditions. Reaction to Prednisone depends on the dosage, with high doses causing more severe side effects. Because my liver functions are so out of whack, I am started on 80 mg per day. Having no previous experience with the drug, I have no expectation of side effects or what this dose means. Within a couple of days, 80 mg of Prednisone daily has turned me into an eating machine with a loathsome attitude. I cannot stop myself from biting Dan's head off every time he walks into the room. I am a harpy—eating us out of house and home—and nasty and short-tempered to boot. But the white spots inside my mouth are disappearing.

Hardly able to stand myself, I decide to read up on the side effects of Prednisone. As with all "miracle" drugs, Prednisone has its drawbacks. Side effects include: weight gain (no kidding), hypertension, diabetes, insomnia, moon face, depression, anxiety, sexual dysfunction, female facial hair growth, balding—*Wait a minute, that's not fair*—osteoporosis or loss of calcium in bones, fatigue, body aches, and sagging skin, among other dreadful effects. *Great. Just great.*

I become very annoyed with my doctor, not an unexpected response since I am furious with the entire world. I struggle through a week of hell. The next liver function test is still elevated but has dropped steeply. I've been through enough. Still very bad-tempered, I decide to taper the Prednisone myself. I'm not going to ask anyone and be told no. A month later, I've tapered myself down to 10 mg per day. I am reconciled with the world—and Dan—and have gotten my face out of the refrigerator.

Another week, I take myself off Prednisone entirely. My liver function tests are near normal and the white spots in my mouth don't return. However, not one of my doctors said, "Gee, your liver functions are looking good, why don't we taper you off the Prednisone?" I doubt that my docs have ever been on daily doses of 80 mg of Prednisone for weeks at a time. Otherwise, I figure, they would know what I've been suffering.

Alright, they deal with life and death issues daily, so maybe my bad attitude or gluttony isn't the most pressing item on their agendas.

I find it ironic that I've experienced both sides of the drug-dose calamity: the catastrophically too rapid taper of dexamethasone that led to a near-psychotic break and the nonexistent, tapering off from Prednisone that threatened to do the same. Where is the common sense in this? And beyond caring for what the patient is going through, there are the economics of these oversights to consider. Untold numbers of ER and urgent care visits could be avoided if drug dosages and resultant side effects were better managed, perhaps even by a phone call from a nurse or pharmacist a couple of days after a prescription was started. A simple, direct outreach call does not strike me as rocket science.

Okay, I'll get off of my soap box now.

After another bone marrow biopsy—*will these ever be over?*—another CT-PET scan, and dozens of blood tests: no trace of cancer. My blood levels are creeping back toward normal. A new healthy me is emerging. This is the outcome for which everyone worked so hard. I am that "new you" that Elspeth happily predicted the day we met Dr. Greyz. My hair is curly, but I have not become Andi McDowell. I revel in my espresso machine, my steadfast husband, my work, home office, and the prints of Paris above my desk. My previous life is back, but not. It might look mostly the same from the outside, but a trickle of joy runs through my days.

DURING THESE LAST MONTHS, I've wondered if Johnny and I can be family. Then a crazy thought occurs to me, *Were we ever family?* Was the environment in which we were raised so stressful, so harmful, as to not qualify as family? I can't answer my own question but remember how growing up we were all expected to sink or swim on our own. Is that what families do? Of course not. That's not the family Dan and I created. We did not make the same disastrous mistakes my parents did. But I wonder if Johnny and I can bridge those deep divides created when we were children; to become a family, perhaps for the first time.

I call and write occasionally, telling Johnny how well I'm doing and thanking him for my new life. Sometimes he answers his phone; sometimes I leave a message that might get returned. I think he's really trying, but we are both clumsy at this family business.

The first Christmas after the transplant, Dan, Elspeth, and I visit him in Willits. It is a cold, gray day. His home is in a neighborhood of small bungalows and a smattering of apartment buildings. Most look cared for and not the scary back street I'd feared. I've never been to Willits and feel out of place. Probably the way Johnny felt in Marin. I'm anxious about inserting myself and my family into his home, his life, and wonder if he feels the same.

Johnny welcomes us with affection. Tacked on the wall are some of the photos I'd mailed him and the Christmas card I'd sent out that year. It's a picture of Johnny and me—with our irrepressible smiles—while I received his stem cell transplant. Below the photo is the word JOY.

There's no Christmas tree, but he's strung colored lights around a living room window. The house is warm. Maybe the ever-hungry geckos that hang out in the huge terrarium in the living room, need the heat. Boxes of cockroaches—gecko food—are lined up against a wall. The fauna makes me uneasy. The house has an earthy smell. I figure it's from Johnny's marijuana plants that he does not show us. I'm also a bit of a clean freak and Johnny's housecleaning is, well, different than mine. But with all of that, Johnny's house has the feel of a place well-loved and cared for.

"What's this?" I ask looking at a complex and colorful wall hanging of abstract animals, geometric patterns, and what appear to be symbols.

"That's my bead work. It's in the style of the Huichol Indians."

"It's gorgeous."

"They take a long time. I wanted to make a business selling them, but I'm not fast enough. Each one takes me weeks."

"Where do you make them?"

"In the garage. It gets pretty cold out there. I give most of them away."

Worried about his comfort and his feet, I ask, "Do you have a rubber mat to stand on?"

Johnny nods. It would be something I would give him if he needed it.

Outside, we meet Buffy and Pepper, and I can see how attached Johnny is to his hens. Walking around the yard, Johnny proudly shows us the well-built chicken coop, the carefully pruned fruit trees, and where his garden will be again this spring.

The four of us walk around the neighborhood. Johnny wears only a tie-dye tee shirt, no jacket. It's in the low forties. The rest of us are freezing. He'd had no jacket last February either so for Christmas I'd bought him some manly, outdoor-type clothing (no tie dye) that might not be his style. I just want to keep him warm.

As the older sister, I am pragmatic and protective and—maybe—too probing, asking him about finding "other" jobs. Even though I do this gently and out of caring, and don't mention illegal substances, Johnny shifts around at my questioning. I know I can't expect my fifty-year-old brother to remake himself simply because I'm concerned about him staying out of jail and having enough money to live on in retirement.

Knowing it's a bad idea, I still ask, "How many quarters do you have in Social Security?"

"I have some. I worked for several years in nursing homes. But maybe not forty."

I feel so stupid. Of course, he doesn't have the minimum forty quarters to qualify for Social Security.

There are other things too that might deepen the divide between us. He mentions an elderly friend of his who has no family. The gentleman lives in Palo Alto and owns a software company in Silicon Valley. He also has a large second home and acreage in the rolling hills to the east of Willits where he invites Johnny to visit. Hearing about this, I inquire in my clumsy and flat-footed manner if he might have written Johnny into his will. He looks at me kindly but as if I've just flunked life. "No, we just sit quietly together. That's what we give each other."

Johnny gives Dan a beaded mandala in the Huichol style; it is a stunning gift.

On the drive home, I worry that my obtuse comments may have had a chilling effect on our relationship, and that makes me sad; but I don't know if I can stop trying to remake and protect my brother. Of course, he doesn't want to be remade, and it's utter hubris on my part to even think that he should. But what might he want and what can I give? Maybe he wants nothing at all. Perhaps I am the one who wants.

# Chapter 60 - Vanity Is the Last to Go

"HEY, PRETTY LADY, you sure have beautiful hair."

I smile at the handsome young African American man who winks at me in the cashier line of a Rite Aid Drug Store.

My hair has grown out, curly for now, as Dr. Greyz predicted. Not brunette, mostly gray, but I have it highlighted and perhaps it suits me.

No longer needing immunosuppressant drugs or Prednisone, my new immune system has accepted its host (me). GVHD has not made a repeat visit.

While I will be vain until the end, there were a couple of moments—while suffering the fevers and chills of septicemia and while being wheeled through the fluorescent underground corridors of the Stanford Hospital in my hated HEPA—that I was so sick and so low that there was no space in my wretched mind for concerns about my appearance. But those were the extremes, and they are over. I still care about how I look.

Since the transplant, my weight has crept back up. I watch what I eat and try to walk three miles a day, but my jeans are snug and don't fit like they used to. B.F.D., right? Another unfortunate remnant of my transplant that titters at my vanity: unwanted facial hair. Yep. At Stanford, I was warned about this unavoidable side effect. The anti-rejection drugs that are a life-saving necessity, cause facial hair growth in women. Probably in men too, but that hardly seems to matter. And the alarmists were right—the anti-rejection medication, and possibly the Prednisone, have caused facial hair. Fine, fuzzy, and prolific. Waxing strips are essential, a good pair of tweezers a must, and with a ten-times magnifying mirror, I can sort of keep things under control.

Nad's are my favorite waxing strips. I like their desensitizing wipes with kava extract. Instructions for their use come in English, Arabic, French, German, Spanish, Italian, Greek, and three other languages I don't recognize. This international product is helping wooly women everywhere. It's the rip heard 'round the world.

In addition to facial hair, the bologna arm infection left a physical mark. The back of my right arm still has a four-inch indentation and a slight darkening along the line of incision.

The final (and I admit miniscule) physical sign of the cancer is the bumpy Hickman. After considerable thought, I decide to have the buried mechanism surgically removed. Given that there'd been a 50-50 chance of it being pulled right out of my chest, I assume that surgical excision would be a quick little slice and a couple of stitches. Wrong. Over the many months that the thingamajig lived in my chest, cartilage had grown around it and encased it in a tough, fibrous capsule. Removal required almost an hour under the knife and was painful. I nearly jumped off the table when the surgeon cauterized an area not sufficiently numbed. Now I have another two-inch scar on my chest, but my décolletage is smooth.

# Chapter 61 - "It Always Comes Back"

*WATCH FOR SYMPTOMS OF Mantle Cell Lymphoma that may indicate a return of the disease:*
- *Swollen lymph nodes*
- *Fever*
- *Night sweats*
- *Loss of appetite*
- *Fatigue*
- *Weight loss*
- *Nausea and/or vomiting*
- *Indigestion*
- *Abdominal pain or bloating*
- *Feeling of fullness*
- *Pressure or pain in lower back, often extending down one or both legs*

Outside of the swollen lymph nodes—and mine might be—I have every symptom on the relapse list. I haven't told Dan and don't want to. My hands shake as I call Dr. Greyz who sends an order for an emergency blood test.

I walk into the lab, where they know me all too well. Leaving the building after the draw, I feel that I am walking backwards into a dream where I was sick. *This can't be happening. I won't let it.* There is something wrong with my left arm. The gauze covering the draw site is soaked with blood, which also runs down to my wrist. I whimper. Bleeding and low platelets are another sign of MCL. I hurry back to the lab. The tech dons a pair of purple latex gloves and removes the bloody gauze.

"Bleeding is a bad sign. I'm so afraid of the test results."

"Aw, Honey. You wait for the numbers. They may be just fine."

The tech cleans up the blood, places a new fold of gauze on my arm, and tapes it down. She looks at me with such compassion that I reach out for her. We put our arms around each other. A man sitting in the reception area smiles and gives me a thumbs up.

Over the past two years since the transplant, I've gotten stronger and healthier and have mostly kept the fear of recurrence out of my thoughts. But as I leave the building a second time, I remember a comment that one of Dan's colleagues made: "It always comes back." Shaking my head, I hum and try to think about dinner, anything but that comment. I want wine. This man's dad died of a relapse, but still, why would he say such a thing to me knowing what I'd been through? Don't people have any sense?

THERE WERE A COUPLE of friends that Dan and I lost over what we thought were brainless, insensitive comments. Steve and Nancy were really Dan's friends from long ago; I'd never been especially close to them. One night shortly after the transplant, Steve launched into a story about a friend of his whose wife had been diagnosed with lymphoma. I tightened at the beginning of this narrative, and Dan and I glanced at each other. Steve went on to say how she was very sick for almost five years and finally died. "But she and my friend had some really good times before she passed away."

I looked at Dan again and could see a fleck of terror in his eyes. I felt it too. What a bizarre story to tell us. Were they trying to assure us that good times were ahead, even if I didn't make it? Thanks anyway.

Later, we had this couple over to our home for dinner during which Nancy regaled us with the same tale. I always thought of Steve as socially challenged, but I was shocked that Nancy would again bring up their unfortunate friend who hád died of lymphoma. What was the point?

But Steve and Nancy weren't done yet. The next—and last—time we got together, Steve, again, brought up the death of this woman. I was close to tears and Dan was angry. How can these people be so crass, so witless, and hurtful?

Dan called the next day to tell Steve that he really hoped they wouldn't bring up this disturbing story again. As Steve was not home, he spoke to Nancy who seemed astonished that what they'd said had been inappropriate. The conversation concluded in neutral territory, but that was the end of our friendship. Steve never called back. I was relieved that I would never again have to brace myself for this retelling of tragedy that cut way too close to the bone.

BUT BACK TO MY FEAR OF a relapse. During a fitful night, I wake repeatedly and go downstairs to check my computer for test results. At 3 AM, they are posted. Low neutrophils and high lymphocytes. Not good. Staring into the blackness outside the window, I wrap my arms around myself. My breaths are quick and shallow. This can't be happening.

The next morning, I get a voice mail from Dr. Greyz.

"I guess you've seen the results of your blood work."

Closing my eyes, I grip the phone. My shoulders rise.

"I've ordered a CT scan for today."

My heart thuds as I tell Dan. He wants to come with me, but I convince him to go to work. I might need him for far more than this trip to the CT trailer.

After another long, fretful night, Dr. Greyz calls with the scan results: no evidence of lymphoma. I phone Dan at work and we both choke back tears of relief. Dr. Greyz says my symptoms must have been a flu. I'm immensely relieved but know that this relapse scare might not be the last, especially for those of us whose malignancies have the nasty habit of a return performance.

If luck is a word one can apply to a grim cancer diagnosis, I am very lucky. While Gael can explain all of the mystifying twists and turns of this illness and my recovery as a sure sign of the work of the Holy Spirit, I am simply grateful to be alive. That I am not disabled or disfigured means so much. I could have easily come out of this like that poor man with the missing face. I still think of him as heroic. Or, like Meera.

There is now the seed of a new idea: I am well and begin to believe that I am free of lymphoma, perhaps for a very long time. It is now up to me to decide what to do with my luminous second chance. Above all, I will not waste it—however I define that.

## Chapter 62 - 2010, Five Years Post-Diagnosis

I RING THE BELL AND MY MOTHER'S caregiver opens the front door. I haven't had a key to my mother's house in years.

The TV blares.

"God that's loud. How do you stand it?" I ask the long-suffering aide.

She shrugs.

"How's Beverly?"

"Won't get out of bed."

"For how long?"

"Four, five days."

I roll my eyes. "Sorry about the extra work and all the noise."

Beverly's caregiver shrugs again. The house is hot and stuffy.

"I'm here," I call walking down the hallway toward the bedroom.

My mother's use of a leather belt on both me and Johnny raised physical welts and left emotional scar tissue. Forty-five years later those memories separate my mother and me more profoundly than geography or life's pressing commitments. Do some marks—like the glaring spots on an x-ray or long, red welts on the back of the legs—change us forever?

We play a mother-daughter charade that at least allows us to see each other a couple of times a year. When we speak, my voice is flat and clipped and has none of the lilt or levity as it does with others.

From her bed, Beverly waves the TV remote at me and turns down the volume. My shoulders relax a bit with the relative quiet. I kiss my mother's cheek. Her arms lift upward in a loose gesture that does not enfold me. I straighten. Beverly glances at the plastic Walgreen's bag I hold.

"I'll pay you."

"My treat."

She nods.

"Do you mind if I open a window?" I ask.

"Oh, don't. I'm always cold."

Putting the back of my hand to my forehead, I wipe upward. My skin feels feverish.

"Can you sit at the vanity?"

"I'm not up to that."

I'm annoyed. No, of course she's not up to that. She's not up to anything except being a housebound victim. I arrange my mother's pillows as Beverly inches toward the middle of the bed. Sitting on the edge, I wrestle with the stiff, heavy plastic and dislodge the pressed powder from its fused cardboard backing.

"Why are these things so impossible to get into?"

"I wish I could help, but… my arthritis. It's not just my knees anymore."

"Do you want to put this on?"

I hold a tortoise-shell hand mirror while Beverly sweeps the ivory face powder onto her still smooth, milky skin. Its floral scent reminds me of the complicated, angry mother I'd known for decades who made up her stunning young face in this same room.

"I'll need you to do the blush and my eyebrows. They're too hard for me."

I hand my mother the mirror. She watches while I brush the rosy, bronze powder onto her cheeks then move my fingertips across her soft, warm face to blend in the color. We are inches from each other. We breathe the same air. The same subdued light grazes our shoulders. The side of my hand rests lightly on my mother's cheekbones as I apply the dusky brown eyebrow pencil. I am unsettled by the arch of her brows, the warmth of her body, her magnolia-white skin. These tiny details remind me of the mother I grew up with, the mother who frightened me, the mother I sometimes hated, and the mother whose love I craved. I finish with the pencil and back away. I turn my face from hers and remember her comment: *You used to be such a pretty girl. I don't know what happened to you.*

"I brought your favorite lipstick."

She expertly applies the Maybelline Craving Coral over her parted lips. She gazes into the mirror then pushes a strand of hair back from her unlined forehead. "A woman's hair is her crowning glory. Mine used to be so nice."

She raises her chin and continues to look at herself. "I wonder how my hair would improve if I didn't have to take all these pain killers." Beverly places the mirror on the bed and clears her throat. "I'm sorry about something."

My eyes remain fixed on the hand mirror.

"I wish I could have done more, you know, when you were sick."

I look up. "That's kind, but we live four hundred miles apart, and you aren't well."

"I know, but...."

"I had Dan and Elspeth and, of course, Johnny."

Beverly's eyes narrow at Johnny's name.

"I don't want to bring up a sore subject. But your son did save my life."

"I don't doubt that."

"So, don't you think he deserves a *little* credit?"

Beverly clasps her hands in her lap. "You weren't around to see what I went through with him."

"Actually, I was. Like the day he came home from the hospital, with no name, remember?"

Now, I'm the one bringing up Johnny.

"He was treated exactly like the rest of you."

"Oh, please. You never held him."

"That's ridiculous."

"You only touched him to hurt him."

"There is so much you don't understand."

"You always say that. It's not true."

*What if I asked her how she berated Johnny every morning at the kitchen table? What if I asked her about putting him outside and leaving him for God knows how long on the swing set in a coat safety-pinned together? She'd deny that it happened. Has she forgotten the chronic and insidious abuse she doled out? The number of times she hit him with a leather belt? Did she forget that she tied him into his crib? What if I reminded her of all that and stormed out the door?*

We'd had this same harangue about Johnny too many times to count. I feel small and stupid for goading my mother. I will not let this conversation happen again. I sigh and say, "I'm sorry. You were being generous, and I turned it into an argument."

Glancing briefly at the TV, Beverly asks, "So, how are you?"

"Fine. I'm working fulltime."

"Really? Are you sure it's not too much?"

"No." I remember the dozens of times my mother said, like today, "*I'm not up to that*," or "*I've overdone it again*," before taking to her bed.

"I like to work."

"You've done well with your life. Much better than I did."

The low jibber-jabber of sales pitches and jingles chirp from the TV. On the screen, a woman caresses a Yoplait yogurt. My heart thumps.

"That's ... that's not true," I say.

But we both know it is. I have done better. Much better. I work; Beverly recuperates but never gets well. I graduated from college; she did not. I married once at thirty-two; Beverly was divorced at thirty-three with four kids. Did I make my choices to be certain that I would never be my mother? Anything but her? *Yes*, likely.

"Oh, it's true." Beverly looks at me then away. "In fact, if you weren't my own daughter, you'd intimidate me."

I lean back and feel as if we are naked. Should I tell my mother that she is ridiculous or embrace her? With one stupefying confession, Beverly has climbed up and peered over the sturdy fortress I've built to protect myself from my mother's rages and disapproval. The emotional bastille I've erected was meant to punish her for being more in love with Vicodin than she seemed to be with Johnny and me, for divorcing my father, for her cruelty, and for her monumental vanity and hypochondria.

While I feel utterly justified in my Alamo approach to my mother, a new thought occurs, *Was it possible—the tiniest bit possible—that I'd not been entirely fair?* Perhaps there was something else I didn't know. Maybe my mother's story was more subtle, more painful, than I understood. Maybe Beverly had tried in ways I didn't see or give her credit for. We sit in an awkward silence.

"My aide is really sick of me. Maybe Johnny would come home and take care of me."

*What?*

I blink. I'm silent, stunned. *Should I laugh?* People are so much deeper than we give them credit for. Maybe they love more than they let on. Or maybe Beverly's memory is shot.

Has she forgotten that she tried for years to get him out of her house? How she asked me, at nineteen, to take him, a thirteen-year-old kid? How she threw him out the day before high school graduation, and now she's thinking he might come back to help her? Is she lucid?

I can't hear any more. I have too much vested in the roles my mother and I have played for so long. If Beverly tries to sweep them away, where would we be? We would lose our equilibrium. We might have to look each other in the eyes, and I am not strong enough for that degree of honesty or intimacy. Not today. Perhaps some other time. Still, there is one thing I give her credit for: she has never said anything really demeaning about my father. Of course, she talked about his drinking and I have sensed hundreds of times that she was bursting to tell me the whole sordid story, but she never did. I have always respected my mother for that.

THE FOLLOWING MONTH Beverly becomes unresponsive and is admitted to a hospital ICU. Dan and I fly south to L.A. and rent a car. When we arrive at the hospital, a young man is attempting to get blood from Beverly's vein. The insides of both her arms are so bruised they appear to bloom with violets. I am angry as the lab tech sticks her again after missing. Beverly's eyes are closed, but she winces. Finally getting the tubes he's after, I say, "No more blood tests. None at all."

The tech looks down. "I'll mention that to the doctor."

"I'm her daughter and I do not want her stuck again."

He nods and leaves the room. Since Beverly had grimaced at the needle sticks, I ask her to squeeze my hand if she can hear me; her brow furrows. Perhaps she is frowning because she can't respond but is trying to. I call her name and ask if she's in pain, or cold, or needs anything. Other than the furrow of her brow, she has no reaction. I wonder if she's afraid.

"Don't worry, we'll be back tomorrow," I tell her.

Early the next morning, Randy, Diane, Dan, and I return to the hospital. While hot outside, the room is air conditioned and I wonder again if Beverly is cold in the thin gown. There's no thermostat in the room. I ask a passing orderly to please bring my mother a warm blanket. Above her bed, the monitors bleep and flash their multi-colored numbers and graphs. We all touch her, call her name, but receive no response. At the nurses' station, I ask if my mother had woken during the night.

"No." The nurse consults a computer screen and tells me that she's been receiving regular doses of morphine and has not been conscious.

"What's wrong with her?"

"Her body is shutting down. It's just her time."

I clutch the edge of the desk and wonder, how does the body simply shut down? I can't understand or accept this. I'm tempted to argue with the nurse but don't. Minutes later, she comes into my mother's room with a syringe.

"Excuse me, what's that?" I ask.

"Morphine."

"Is it necessary?"

"We don't want your mother to be in pain."

"Nor do we, but she doesn't appear to be in any distress."

"This will ensure her comfort."

I am not going to raise an issue but think this extra narcotic doesn't seem right. While I have begun to accept that this is the end for my mother, I don't see the need to keep pumping her with morphine, except to move things along. But this situation is out of my league. While I'd advocated for myself for conscious sedation, here I'm uncertain of the issues and even about what is best for my mother. I resent the rush, as much for Beverly, as for myself.

After administering the morphine, the nurse removes the oxygen mask.

*What has just happened that Beverly doesn't need oxygen anymore?*

Under the mask, her mouth, cheeks, and chin are caked with dried blood and mucous. She looks so shockingly bad that I groan. At the small sink in her room, I pour warm water onto a paper towel and begin gently wiping at her cheeks where the blood is a fine red skein over her skin. Lying back, her face is creaseless, and she looks much younger than her eighty-three years. I finish washing my mother's cheeks and clean her bloody chin. But her mouth and lips are sticky with blood and yellow mucous that makes me queasy. I soak a new paper towel and gently start to remove the disgusting ooze that has collected. I don't want to get the awful stuff on my hands. Again and again, I go back for more damp paper. While I might have called a nurses' aide to remove the slime from my mother's mouth, I need to do it myself. After Beverly is clean, I wash my hands with hot soapy water then dab a bit of perfume on her neck from a tiny bottle of Hawaiian umé I carry in my purse; not the Shalimar she always wore, but still.

Dan and Randy go to the cafeteria for coffee. Diane answers phone calls in the hallway. I watch the monitors. Beverly's breathing and pulse are slowing. A heavy lunch cart rumbles past the door. Dan brings me coffee and I put my hands around the warm cardboard, remembering the pleasure I found in my morning latte while I was in the hospital. My mother's pulse rate slows further. Diane finishes her calls. A man groans from another room.

The nurse comes back and stands with the four of us. Only the quiet, rhythmic mechanical beeping breaks the silence. We watch the monitors as they register progressively less activity.

"I'm afraid she's gone," says the nurse.

"But there's still movement," I answer.

"The machine will shut down shortly."

"How do you know?"

"Your mom has passed."

I stare at the nurse who says, "I'm sorry."

My chin drops to my chest, and a primal keen rises from my center. Then come wracking sobs, my shoulders and chest heave. Dan holds me, then Randy, then Diane; everyone comforts me. The intensity of my response shocks me, not because I didn't love my mother, I did; but I am not expecting this. In these moments of hard grieving, after she dies, I feel like Beverly's daughter—a role that has never been natural or easy. There will be no reconciliation now.

My body still shakes as Dan wraps his arms around me. We are quiet, all of us gazing at Beverly for some minutes. I inhale a big, shuddering breath. Then, an idea occurs to me.

I ask Dan, "Will you take a picture of me and Randy with Beverly?"

Randy's eyes widen and he looks at me as if I've had some sort of lapse.

"I know it's a bit weird, but it also feels respectful, important, even loving."

Randy agrees and we hover around her bed, the two of us leaning inward. Beverly does not appear peaceful, just disinterested, gone. Randy looks so much like our father in these pictures—the graying goatee and mustache, the solemn piercing gray eyes, the set mouth. As if our father had come back for this moment. I smile, a sad little smile. I feel lost, orphaned. The monitors no longer glow with numbers; our electronic assurances have ceased. The room is perfectly quiet. I kiss my mother's still warm face and touch her hand.

Randy and Diane say goodbye to her then leave to make arrangements for a family-only memorial dinner at their home. Dan and I stay with Beverly while we wait for the undertakers. I smell the perfume on my fingers.

"Did I ever tell you about my mother and the hula skirt?" I ask.

Dan smiles and shakes his head, "No."

"I was maybe nine. It was the night before Halloween. Beverly was out with a girlfriend. I'd put the boys to bed and was trying to make a Hawaiian skirt for my costume by sewing blue and green streamers of crepe paper onto a cotton waistband. But the paper tore over and over and I kept sticking the needle into my fingers. I was frustrated and sad that I wouldn't have a costume. But I just couldn't do it and gave up. I left Beverly a note asking that she please help me. The next morning, I opened my eyes and heard the sewing machine and the rustling of crepe paper."

"That's a good memory. I'm glad you told me."

"The rustling of that paper was the most beautiful sound I'd ever heard."

The undertakers arrive, and I kiss my mother for the last time. They move Beverly onto a gurney, and wheel her out of the ICU. As we watch her go, I am thankful that—washing her face—the last kindness she received had been from me. I'm glad I remembered the hula skirt story to tell Dan.

Randy and Diane do not want my help with dinner. Getting only answering machines, I make a few phone calls to friends and family letting them know about Beverly's passing. I call Johnny and leave a message on his machine. Same with Tom, who I'd been calling for two days. Diane urges me to take care of myself and suggests I gets a pedicure. The idea strikes me as odd, but anything I might have done that afternoon would have been odd.

It is a stifling July afternoon and the air-conditioned salon in the corner of the hot, dusty strip mall is empty. As my feet soak in the warm, scented water, I close my eyes and question if the affection I'd shown my mother in cleaning her face was also an act of forgiveness.

But perhaps it is arrogance to think that I should be forgiving her. If Beverly could have spoken in these last two days, would she have told me that she was sorry? Would she have admitted to doing a terrible job as a mother?

Or would I have heard a story about her life that was far different from the one I thought I knew?

I am trying to state these questions as clearly as I can, but the answers are not simple or obvious. Just the month before, my mother had startled me with the intimate confession of her perceived inadequacy. Beverly had never shared that sort of feeling before. Perhaps she felt it was important for me to know her better, to open up an avenue of discussion, to be honest with each other before it was too late. Did she have an inkling that the conversation couldn't wait? What do we perceive about our own deaths? I'd asked the same question when my father died and am no closer to having an answer.

I don't hear back from Johnny. Tom doesn't pick up my call for several days. We have our memorial service without them.

# Chapter 63 - Loving Doesn't Have to Be Close Up

IT'S 2020. DAN AND I ARE RETIRED. In 2016, we bought a new house, my dream house. It's a concrete and glass, Mid-Century Modern. Not for everyone, but we both love this place. It's about a mile as the crow flies from our last place; we still live on the edge of the San Francisco Bay.

I've told him that this is the home I will be carried out of, feet first. With only a touch of irony, I've already shown him where, in the living room, I want my hospital bed and how close the Sauvignon Blanc and the morphine should be.

As many times as people have said, "You have been so strong throughout your cancer ordeal." I never *felt* strong. I've accomplished a few things in my life that were very hard for me: Attending U.C. Berkeley and finishing a degree in Public Health and Immunology. Every day I felt incompetent and wanted to drop out, but I kept pushing ahead and got that diploma. Quitting cigarettes was a real test of will; but I did that too. And breastfeeding Elspeth for the first two weeks was so painful that I cried as much as she did. Still, I would not give up, and eventually we got it right. These things were *hard* for me and required every fleck of grit and determination I could muster. "Fighting" cancer was different. It required that I show up and cooperate, endure some pain, and occasionally excuse ineptitude.

Being a survivor has made me realize that there isn't time to beat myself up for real or perceived deficiencies, or wallow around in negativity. The ticking of the clock has a new trace of urgency, but it is a fine thing. It is not worrisome. Instead, it feels as if two hands are behind me, gently pushing me forward in a helpful, encouraging manner, enabling me to maintain a gratifying forward momentum.

Enduring the biopsies, the chemo, the sepsis, and the transplant created a stronger, less neurotic me. Grace was born amidst the suffering brought on by Mantle Cell Lymphoma, and that grace quieted the howl of my childhood terrors of chaos, abandonment, and feeling unloved. I can now reject the rant of inadequacy that bellowed inside me since childhood. I no longer run from a damning voice; I move now because I have strong legs and lungs and a lot of ground to cover.

What I don't have any more—and miss them—are the visions I had during my illness. The beauty of the sky as it trembled, or feeling the earth breathe, or colors quiver. Nothing separated me from that which was not me. We—it—were all one thing. One perfect thing.

I've read passages by writers who described death—or a near death experience—and the similarities to my visions astound me—loss of ego, merging of the spiritual self with that outside the body, peace, tranquility, and overwhelming wonder.

I've not seen these miraculous visions since my recovery. Or any pink clouds around my bed.

I often think of Johnny. Our bond was built on history and gratitude, but these did not prove strong enough to hold together the two vastly different people we had become, or perhaps always were. I do not stop wanting to protect him, but never know how, except by being strong, capable, and ultimately distant. While I sometimes wish there was a profound way to repay him, I now understand that all I can give him is my love and concern and the occasional financial leg up. And this is okay for both of us. Loving doesn't have to be close up. Sometimes it can't be.

## Chapter 64 - Forgiveness Is a Lifetime, Not a Moment

I WALK DOWN MY CLEAN, well-landscaped street and reach the north end of the San Francisco Bay. It is summer. Eleven years ago today my mother died. And more than fourteen years ago I received my stem cell transplant. Maybe, like the woman said at the Center for Attitudinal Healing, it is nonsense to think we will all die of our cancers.

Today the Bay is a great bowl of green, silver, and blue water. Small, ceaseless waves from the broad horizon break up and down the beach. The massive freighters—heading west, out the Golden Gate—unleash their deep blast waves that rumble through me. I breathe in the salt air that streams off the bay and blows the hair away from my face.

Sitting on a flat stone, I am struck by the irony: my mother had her thunderous morality and strict Catholicism, my father had his tough guy, Mad Men persona; yet I'm the strong one. And even with my history of lymphoma, I will always be the healthy one.

I've been trying for years to sort all of this out. It will not be sorted. It just is and all I can do is accept it.

I remember what Johnny said, "I've spent a lot of my life fighting my way out of the darkness of my childhood, but I finally understand that it's impossible to expect love or compassion from someone living in hell."

Johnny has no animosity for Mom or Dad. Why do I still blame them for their cruelty and abandonment, if he doesn't? I don't know the answer to that question. Perhaps I should try harder to forgive.

People who are religious might cheer, "Shout it out, Sister, and welcome God into your heart."

I remove my sandals, roll up my jeans, and reach into a small daypack. First, I pull out a blue velvet string bag—about the size of a child's fist—then a bouquet of eight ranunculus, all orange except for one red flower. The content of the tiny bag is what remains from my mother's cremation.

Looking out over the Bay, I whisper to my parents, "See where I live? Isn't it beautiful?"

Walking across the gritty sand, I am soon calf-deep in the cold, swirling water. I open the bag and sprinkle a small bit of ash onto the restless current. I release the bouquet. The ashes and the flowers are pulled out with the receding wave. The blossoms bob on the surface and are then submerged. Some reappear. With each retreating wave, another flower disappears; now there are two orange blooms and the red one. I watch until all of the flowers have been taken out to sea. The papery red ranunculus is the last to disappear.

I press the velvet bag to my heart. I close my eyes and listen to the surging water. Will I ever be able to make the simple but profound decision to forgive my parents? That sounds like hubris and maybe it is. Still, I murmur, "I'll try. I promise, I'll try."

# Author's Postscript

IN 2005-2006, WHILE HOSPITALIZED for a lymphoma I was not expected to survive, I kept a hit-or-miss journal. In 2012, I transcribed those thirty pages and began to fill in the blanks. I also culled material from my medical record—all 1,210 pages of it! Docs write the most amazing and revealing things in their patient notes. Over the next few years, this memoir began to take shape.

I wasn't certain why I was writing, but the further into it I got, the more I knew I had to keep going. The manuscript grew, and I began to understand that the writing—along with chemo, radiation, and the bone marrow transplant—was also an avenue to healing.

It began to dawn on me that I had been struggling with two disorders: the cancer as well as the aftermath of a traumatizing childhood. I was never good enough for my parents; so, as an adult, I had to prove my worth with academic, career, and financial achievements. And even when chemo had beaten me into a bilious haze, I could rarely give myself a morning or afternoon off. From my hospital bed, I still handled as much work as I could. I've joked that my tombstone will read, *The last item on Susan's To-Do List.*

Much research points to early childhood trauma as a risk factor for both physical and psychological disorders: from adult depression to post-traumatic stress disorder (PTSD) and most other psychiatric illnesses, as well as cardiovascular disease, cancer, and obesity. While I endured a violent childhood, I cannot claim with any certainty that the trauma of my early years led to malignancy. Depression, yes. Compulsivity, definitely. A tendency to rely on alcohol too heavily, probably. Cancer, well, who knows?

Whatever the cause of my lymphoma, my obsession to write about that extraordinary year of treatment and to accomplish something concrete in those otherwise drifting, aimless months, is where I trust my compulsivity will benefit others.

My goal in writing *Blood Brother* is that it will bring hope to those who face the grimmest diagnoses. My story proves that life can be shockingly kind and generous. The odds can be beaten.

While memories from my childhood are mine alone and recollections from the months in the hospital while undergoing treatment may have been colored by the hefty number of drugs I was taking, the events reported in this memoir are accurate. I've relayed every detail of my childhood, illness, and recovery with the utmost honesty, respect, and love.

Thank you for joining me on this journey.

Stay safe. Be well.

# Simple Ideas for a Better Hospital Stay

YEARS AGO, DAN WAS SENT to Honolulu on a business trip, and I tagged along. One evening, we attended a wine and cheese reception hosted by the hotel where we were guests. The manager of the hotel approached me and asked about our stay, which had been lovely. Then he asked if there was anything else that I could suggest as an improvement. The question was simple and I had an immediate answer. "Yes, on the automated wake-up call don't have the recorded voice say, 'Good Morning'; have the voice say, 'Aloha.'" We *were* in Hawaii, for goodness sake! He looked at me as if I was brilliant, but my suggestion was so simple that it seemed obvious. Sometimes we are just too close to see how to improve.

The list below contains a few of those simple little suggestions that might improve the quality of a patient's stay and even perhaps enhance their clinical and quality-of-life outcomes.

- When patients leave the hospital, put a printed note card in their bag of take-home meds. The note could read, "You're a Champ!" and be signed by the hospital staff (rubber stamp signatures are fine). Or "We're happy to partner with you," or another expression of comradery and support. Of equal importance, include a phone number for the floor's nurses' station in case the patient has a follow-up question.

- A card in the patient's room with the offerings of the Espresso cart! Oh, how I would have loved to have known about the espresso cart a lot earlier. Also, if the patient is not capable of walking, the coffee could be brought to the patient's room with a small service fee tacked onto the hospital bill.

- A nurse offering a simple cookie or biscuit with coffee or juice after colonoscopy, endoscopy, or other procedure in which fasting is required.

- A small notepad in each patient room along with a pen. On each page of the notepad, could be printed: If You Like, Write Down Three Things You are Grateful for Today.

- An Outreach Rx call. I suffered terribly from withdrawal of dexamethasone and no taper of Prednisone. Had a nurse or pharmacist called to check up on me, they might have been able to better taper my meds and keep me from the emotional shattering I endured. This sort of outreach can also prevent numerous and unnecessary ER and urgent care visits, thus saving the system money.

- Instruct employees that "No problem," is not an appropriate response when a patient says, "Thank you," especially in a hospital environment where there tends to be plenty of problems!

- In institutions that *will not* offer conscious sedation for painful procedures, such as bone marrow biopsies and aspirations, consider offering patients a bit of fentanyl, perhaps like that contained in a sucker. Even if it is little more than a placebo-sized dose, it might help with the pain, and the gesture will likely be appreciated.

- How about improving the décor with a little more color or cheerful photographs?

- While it is not a small change, I enthusiastically applaud the role that Nurse Navigators are now taking to make the patient experience so much better. How I wish I would have had a Nurse Navigator as my go-to person during my many hospital stays.

- Fifteen years on, I still receive treatment several times a year for infusion of antibodies. My immune system, while active and protective, gets fatigued every few months and needs a booster. When I check into the Oncology Infusion Area, the lovely gentleman at the desk always knows my name. His, "Good morning, Susan," makes me feel welcome and cared for. The trust this instills in me is amazing. While this might be difficult in a busy hospital, use people's names whenever possible. If names are too much to expect, a smile will go a long way to making patients feel welcomed and relaxed.

- I loved that my hospitalist, Dr. Arent, dressed up as Big Bird for Halloween. Consider a bit of humor wherever possible.

- Like the manager of the Honolulu hotel asked me, ask patients, "Is there anything we could do to make your visits easier for you?"

# Acknowledgements

To my wonderful fellow writers and editors: John Byrne-Barry, Katherine Ellison, Molly Giles, Jo Haraf, Laura Hilgers, Jonathan Krim, Barbara Linkevitch, Jean Mansen, Stefanie Marlis, Elspeth Scott, and Tommie Whitener. To my ace proofreader, Arnetta Jackson.

To my early readers: Nancy Andrews, RN, Mimi Choi, MD, Candy delPortillo, Amy Ewing, MD, Natalya Greyz, MD, Barbara Holbert, Meryl Luallin, Gael Milner, RN, Molly Porter, Linda Toy, and Jessica Wimer, RN.

To those of you who helped me every step of the way: Sally Arai, MD, Laurie and Richard Favaro, Jeanne and Dennis Garro, Michael and Christina Gleason, Carl Hart, Susan Keane-Baker, Suzy Loughlin, Gael and Tony Milner, Anne and Will Mosgrove, Randy and Diane Shultz, and Lori Smith.

To Jenn Haskin, my terrific editor—thanks for your wisdom, spot-on suggestions, and incredible support—and to Sheri Williams, publisher at TouchPoint Press, who took a chance on me.